The Minimalist Natural Medicine Cabinet

The Minimalist Natural Medicine Cabinet

Creating a Small Collection of Remedies
to Meet Common Household Needs

Kristen Smith

Herbalist & Aromatherapist

The Minimalist Natural Medicine Cabinet

Kristen Smith, ABetterWayToThrive.com

Cover and interior photo by Kiki Siepel (https://unsplash.com/photos/BEwxLSN_bKU) on Unsplash.

ISBN: 979-8-9859050-0-7 (print)

ISBN: 979-8-9859050-1-4 (e-book)

Table of Contents

Part 1: Introduction 1

  Does It Have to Be So Complicated? 2
  Let's Simplify Things 4
  The Minimalist Natural Medicine Cabinet.....................5
  How Natural Health Works 6
  How to Use This Book 11

Part 2: The Remedies 15

  Aloe Gel 18
  Apple Cider Vinegar..20
  Arnica 22
  Baking Soda..24
  Bentonite Clay 25
  Carrier Oil..26
  Cold & Flu Relief Tea...28
  Echinacea Extract..31
  Elderberry Syrup or Gummies 34
  Epsom Salt..37
  Essential Oils 38
  Garlic 46
  Ginger..49
  Healing Salve..52
  Honey 55
  Lemon..57
  Relaxing Nervine Tea 59
  Sea Salt..62
  Tummy Tea..64
  Turmeric 67
  Witch Hazel...70

Part 3: Common Ailments 73

  Acne/Blemishes...76
  Allergies (Seasonal) 77

Bruises, Sprains, & Strains 78

Bug Bites & Stings 79

Burns 80

Constipation 81

Coughs 83

Cuts & Scratches 85

Diarrhea 86

Dry Skin 87

Earaches 88

Fatigue 90

Fever 92

Fungal Skin Infections (Tinea Infections) 94

Gas & Bloating 96

Growing Pains 98

Headaches 99

Heartburn & Indigestion 101

Immune System Support 103

Insomnia & Restlessness 104

Joint Pain 105

Menstrual Cramps 107

Muscle Pain 109

Nasal & Sinus Congestion 110

Nausea & Upset Stomach 112

Poison Ivy/Oak/Sumac 114

Rashes 116

Sore Throat 118

Stress & Anxiety 120

Teething 121

Warts 122

Part 4: Continued Learning 123

Final Encouragement 124

Let's Connect 125

One-on-One Help 126

Keep Learning with Additional Resources 127

Acknowledgments 12/

About the Author 129

Part 1:
Introduction

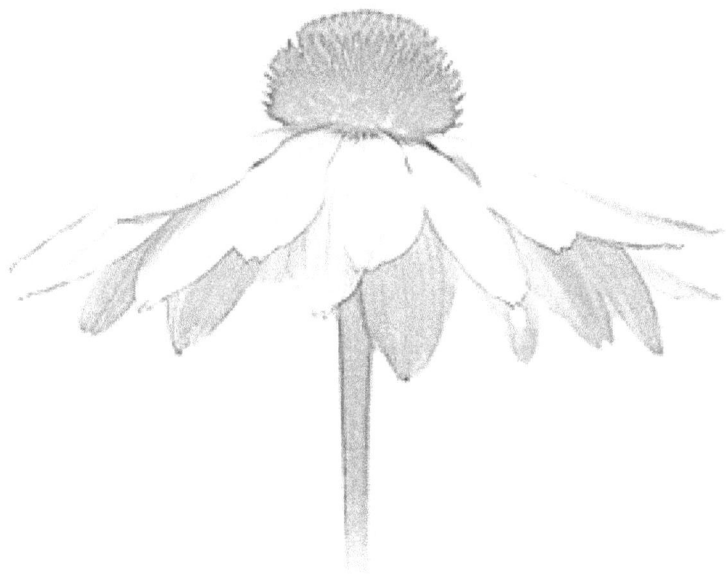

Does It Have to Be So Complicated?

Shortly after my husband and I were married, I decided to make an apple pie since he loved the ones my mom made.

But this wasn't going to be just any apple pie. *This* pie was going to have a beautiful, homemade lattice crust. Not only that, I was also going to use less sugar and leave the apples unpeeled to make it a more sensible dessert for the two of us.

It was a great plan. Except, I had never made a pie, let alone a reduced-sugar, lattice-crust unpeeled apple pie.

I still remember how frustrated I was as my lattice strips broke and crumbled while I tried to weave them together. I looked like a 6-year-old learning to tie his shoes and felt like it, too.

When we were eating it, I ventured to ask my husband what he thought of the pie. There was a pause.

"Your mom just makes really good pie, honey," he broke the news to me.

Though I laugh about it now, he was right. I took on a project far too advanced for my skills and we ended up with some rather underwhelming results.

Unfortunately, this same type of scenario happens to many people when they get started with natural remedies.

They're excited, maybe even a little ambitious. They're ready to completely overhaul their medicine cabinet and replace everything with natural options.

They dive into internet research, fill up their Pinterest boards, and maybe even hit the library for real books.

But then their heads start spinning with all the information. It seems like there are so many remedies to buy and things to make.

Not to mention worrying about safety, time commitments, and storing it all.

Before long, they feel so in over their heads that they decide this natural remedy stuff is best left to the experts, or at least the folks with way more experience than they have.

If this sounds at all familiar to you, I have good news for you.

You're not alone.

And I propose a better way.

Let's Simplify Things

A natural medicine cabinet can actually be surprisingly simple.

While herbalists and aromatherapists like me may stock their home apothecaries with dozens, perhaps even hundreds, of herbs, extracts, essential oils, and other remedies, you'll probably only need a small fraction of that.

You see, there are likely thousands of medicinally valuable plants and remedies. Some of them are quite specific, exotic, or rare.

But others can meet numerous needs, so you don't need to have hundreds of specific remedies on hand. They're often very safe, too. Because of this, they've earned reputations as must-haves and are easy to find.

These are the remedies that deserve a spot in your medicine cabinet.

This small collection of versatile, easy to find remedies can work very well for most people. I like to think of this as the Minimalist Natural Medicine Cabinet.

The Minimalist Natural Medicine Cabinet

A Minimalist Natural Medicine Cabinet is all about making natural remedies more affordable, more accessible, and less intimidating.

Stocking a large collection of remedies can cost quite a bit of money, especially when some of those remedies aren't your everyday backyard herb.

Large home apothecaries require specialty purchases or extensive gardening and/or production skills in order to get all the remedies. But not everyone wants to or is able to devote all the money, time, and space for that.

Even more so, expansive natural remedy collections demand you actually know how to use all of those remedies. And that's often the most intimidating factor of all.

However, when you stock a small but effective collection of remedies, you'll bypass these roadblocks.

You'll develop a deep understanding of a few remedies instead of a broad familiarity with many. You'll spend less money by buying less and are more likely to see better results with the money you've spent. Finally, you'll gain experience with the natural approach to health and wellness that will snowball to greater confidence and success.

In time, you'll be able to add more specialty remedies to your medicine cabinet if you need or want to. But in the beginning, simplicity works to your advantage.

Just like I needed to stick to a basic apple pie recipe.

How Natural Health Works

Before we dive into what goes on the shelves of a Minimalist Natural Medicine Cabinet, it's important to pause a moment and talk about how natural health best works.

In our quick-fix, pop-a-pill culture, it's understandable that you might assume natural remedies work the same way.

Have a headache? No problem! Instead of ibuprofen or acetaminophen, just take this herbal capsule of wonders and your headache will disappear in under half an hour.

Runny nose? Here, just use these essential oils to dry up the drip and be sniffle-free for the rest of the day.

Kids running a fever? Bring that temperature down with this extract and get back to your regular program in no time.

It's a good thing natural health doesn't work that way.

Allow me to explain.

Prevention is Key

The adage "an ounce of prevention is worth a pound of cure" is a common phrase because there's so much truth in it. It's generally much easier to prevent an illness than it is to treat it.

In natural health, the goal is to prevent illnesses from happening in the first place. Not only is this easier, but it also simplifies your remedy stash. The more illnesses you can prevent, the fewer remedies you need.

As you're building your natural medicine cabinet, you should also reflect on your entire approach to health. This isn't about complicated diets or expensive supplement protocols, though.

We're talking simple:

- How much sugar, white flour, and hydrogenated oils do you regularly eat?
- How many fresh or frozen vegetables and fruits do you eat every day?
- How much water do you drink daily?
- How many times a week do you get in healthy activity and movement?
- How much sleep do you get every night?
- How would you rate your stress levels?

Of course, you can never hold off sickness completely. Even the most dedicated, all-organic, all-natural, super-fit person in the world is likely to come down with a cold now and then.

But keying in on your overall diet, lifestyle, and health habits can go a long way in keeping you healthy. And when you do get sick, your body will have the strength and reserves it needs to fight off the infection more easily.

Look for Root Causes

Finding root causes is another foundation of natural health. These help you better understand why you got sick so you can address that need and protect against sickness in the future.

Let's use the common cold as an example.

With a conventional mindset, you might come down with a cold and assume you just picked up the cold virus somewhere. Your body had to succumb to it and it's all that virus's fault for invading you.

With a holistic health mindset, you retrace your recent habits, stress levels, diet, and such after you get sick. You might even ask yourself some of the same questions from the section above to uncover why your body wasn't able to fight off the cold virus this time.

Usually, it's easy to figure out the root causes of a short-term illness. These often happen after holidays or periods of extended stress when your diet, sleep, and other lifestyle habits suffer.

Finding the root causes of chronic conditions is more complicated and often requires the help of an integrative healthcare provider or natural health practitioner. It's still worth investigating, though, as finding those root causes can help unlock deeper healing.

Sometimes a root cause isn't obvious, and that's okay. There's no need to stress over finding one if you simply came down with a cold. But it's always worth considering anytime you get sick or have another health concern.

Looking for root causes is never about one thing, though. And that's guilt or blame. Blaming yourself for sickness, whether your own or someone else's, will only add more stress and make it more difficult to heal. When you uncover a root cause, be ready to let go of any disappointment you may feel in yourself or others. Learn what you can, then move forward.

Work with Symptoms

Conventional over-the-counter remedies typically work by taking away uncomfortable symptoms. Of course, this isn't always a bad thing. No one enjoys headaches, runny noses, or fevers. Sometimes you have to remove symptoms in the short term so overall healing can take place.

But too often, conventional remedies mask or remove symptoms and stop there. Consider this common scenario.

Your child wakes up not feeling well, and within a few hours, her temperature rises to 100.4°F. You know the fever isn't dangerous, but she's uncomfortable. Not wanting her to suffer and hoping to curb the illness, you grab the children's liquid ibuprofen and give her indicated doses throughout the day.

By nightfall, her fever is gone, but other symptoms of the infection linger off and on for a couple of weeks. You treat them as they arrive: cough medicine to stop the coughs, nasal decongestant to unplug her nose, and finally, an antibiotic to clear up the ear infection that set in two weeks later.

Six weeks go by, and the same cycle repeats with the same predictable results.

On the surface, it appears these treatments all helped her recover from the illness, even though she got sick again shortly after.

But did they? Or did they only take away the symptoms and mask the deeper needs?

Consider what the above scenario might look like through the lens of natural health.

Your child comes down with a fever and shows signs of illness. She's uncomfortable, so you encourage her to lie down and place a cool cloth on her forehead for comfort. You make her a cup of Cold & Flu tea and she sips it over the course of an hour. The tea makes her sweat a little, keeping her fever at a more comfortable level.

You start dosing elderberry syrup to give her immune system a boost at fighting off the infection. When she starts coughing, you encourage her to keep drinking her tea and add a little honey and ginger to it to soothe her throat. When her nose gets stuffy, you apply a safe essential oil blend, properly diluted, to her chest and neck to help break up the congestion.

She drinks the Cold & Flu tea for three days and takes elderberry syrup for seven. But by the end of five days, she's completely back to normal except for a slight runny nose. At the end of the week, her symptoms are gone and her illness is resolved.

In the first example, you help your child feel better in the short term by taking away her symptoms, but her body ends up sicker. In the second, you give your child some comfort measures while letting her symptoms work towards healing.

The body usually knows what it's doing with those symptoms.

Support the Body's Healing Mechanisms

Similar to the previous point, a final goal of natural health is to support the body's own healing processes. While this seems like a common sense thing to do, it isn't always so obvious.

Sometimes, these healing mechanisms look like sickness, as in the case of fevers and runny noses. These symptoms are sometimes annoying or uncomfortable, but they have an important job to do.

Consider fevers, for instance. Fevers make our bodies less hospitable to pathogenic microbes. When a fever is allowed to do its work, the invading microbes can be weakened, attacked, and removed from the body more quickly.

But when a fever is suppressed, the body's intelligent response to an invader is stopped. The infecting microbes get the advantage and the illness may end up lasting longer or becoming more complicated in the end.

That's not to say that you should never try to lower a fever or intervene when the body is reacting to something. But before stepping in to stop a symptom, ask yourself if that symptom could be the body's way of restoring health and encouraging a smart, finely-tuned immune system.

As you continue through this book, keep these goals in mind. Start to shift your thinking to a more holistic way of looking at sickness, one that

- Emphasizes prevention.
- Looks for root causes.
- Works with symptoms, instead of masking them.
- And supports the body's own healing mechanisms.

You might find that mindset is the most important thing you can add to your medicine cabinet!

How to Use This Book

Now that we have some important groundwork laid, it's time to start developing your Minimalist Natural Medicine Cabinet.

In the following pages, you'll find two main sections: one dedicated to remedies, and one dedicated to common household ailments.

You can use this book as a simple reference book, turning to it when needs arise. But you'll be better prepared for those needs and likely get more out of the coming pages if you go through them in order at least once.

The Remedies

It was a fun challenge to keep the list of remedies as concise as possible. As an herbalist and aromatherapist, I have so many "favorite" herbs that it almost felt like I was choosing friends for an elementary dodgeball team. Thankfully, herbs and remedies don't have feelings, so those that were cut can still hold a special place in my personal medicine cabinet.

When looking at possible remedies, I focused on four important qualifications. To make the list, the remedy had to be

- Versatile: helpful in multiple situations.
- Effective: produce reliable results.
- Safe: free from potentially serious side effects.
- Convenient: relatively easy to find, store, and administer.

You'll find herbs, essential oils, kitchen ingredients, and general first aid products in the remedy list.

You won't find many homeopathic remedies, though. I include one, but homeopathy is a modality quite different from herbalism and aromatherapy and one I don't use often in my home and herbal practice. If you're interested in stocking your medicine cabinet with homeopathic remedies, it's important to understand the philosophy behind homeopathy and how it differs from other healing modalities.

Before you worry that you'll have to DIY everything as you build your arsenal of natural remedies, fear not. I've included both buying tips and recipes, so you can decide if you want to make something or purchase it.

I've also set up a special list on my Amazon Storefront with examples of the remedies you might like to buy. You can purchase through the storefront or use it to help you make other purchases.

The Ailments

The next section includes common household ailments and potential remedies you can use to overcome them. Like the previous section, they're listed in alphabetical order.

Along with options from the previous remedy list, I've included additional remedies that are specific to that particular ailment.

For example, if you are prone to coughs, colds, and lung congestion, I suggest mullein leaf (*Verbascum thapsus*) as an herb that can help strengthen your respiratory system and promote clearer breathing. Mullein leaf didn't make the cut for the Minimalist Natural Medicine Cabinet, but it's my top pick for respiratory concerns.

When you look up ways to treat an ailment, you can refer back to the list of remedies for detailed information on dosing and administration.

When to Seek Medical Advice

Finally, it's important to remind you that I am not a licensed healthcare provider. The following information is for educational use and is not a substitute for medical advice. You alone are responsible for how you use natural remedies in your home.

Never hesitate to seek medical care if an illness isn't responding to natural remedies, seems to worsen, or your intuition tells you that you need more expert care.

Conventional medical treatment can handle life-threatening, serious, and acute health situations quickly and powerfully. There is no shame in using that care if it offers the most reliable, needed results.

That said, most common home ailments can be safely treated at home with simple remedies. Let's move on and take a look at those remedies now.

Part 2:
The Remedies

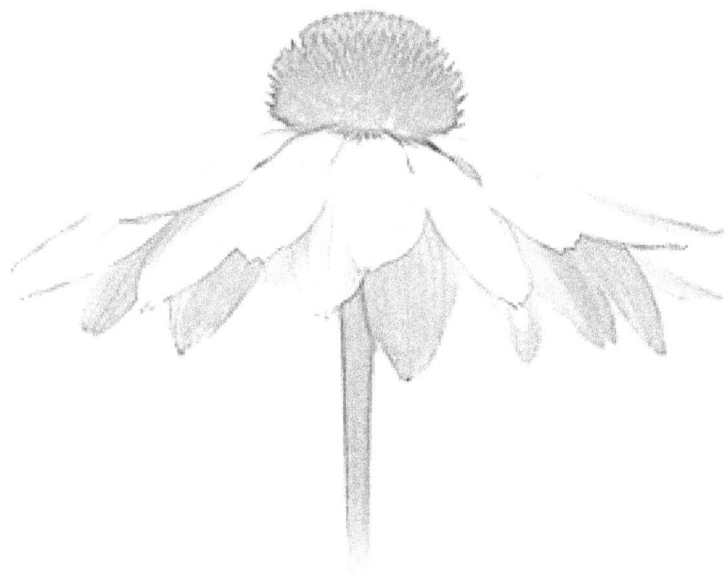

As mentioned in the previous section, the following remedies meet four important qualifications: they're safe, effective, versatile, and convenient. The entries are listed in alphabetical order and include the following helpful information:

- **Where to Find** helps you know if you can find the remedy at a supermarket, health food store, or online specialty supplier.
- **What to Look for When Buying** gives you tips on choosing quality products.
- **Shelf Life** gives you guidance on how long your remedies will last, as well as storage tips.
- **Actions** explains what the remedy does and how it works.
- **Preparations** shares how you can use the remedy, such as in a tea, compress, or bath. **Dosage** information is given where applicable.
- **Contraindications** gives important safety information, especially when it comes to children and pregnant or breastfeeding women.
- **How to Make** gives you instructions on how to make your own remedy, when applicable.

To make it even easier for you to see examples of the remedies, and even buy them if you choose, I've created a special protocol on my Wellevate online dispensary called Minimalist Natural Medicine Cabinet. Wellevate allows you to shop high-quality and professional-grade herbal products, dietary supplements, person care products, and more.

The products included in the Minimalist Natural Medicine Cabinet protocol are excellent options you can consider as you stock your remedies. To see the list:

1. Visit my Wellevate online dispensary: https://wellevate.me/kristen-smith-1
2. Click on the protocol labeled "Minimalist Natural Medicine Cabinet."
3. Scroll through the items I included. You can purchase through the dispensary and even shop for other professional-grade supplements at 15% off while you're there.

I've included comments for each item, so look for the little description by every listing to learn more.

For herbal projects, you can find links to reputable ingredient providers here: https://abetterwaytothrive.com/recommended-products.

Aloe Gel

Aloe gel is made from the internal pulp of the *Aloe vera* plant and is used for burns and dry, injured, or irritated skin.

Where to Buy

Aloe gel is available from most drugstores, grocery stores, and other big box stores, but watch for preservatives and other added ingredients. The best quality will come from herbal supply stores, health food stores, or Wellevate. The simplest way to have the purest form of aloe gel at the ready is to keep an aloe plant in your home.

Buying Tips

Look for aloe gel that is free from artificial colors and fragrances. Most aloe gels contain a minute amount of stabilizers, thickening agents, and/or preservatives. Quality aloe gels are over 99% aloe. Purchase only enough aloe gel that you can use up within a year.

Shelf Life

Depending on how much preservative is included with your aloe, the shelf life may be anywhere from 1 year to many years. Quality aloe gels, with minimal preservatives, will last around 1 year and are best kept refrigerated.

Actions

- *Emollient*—soothes and protects damaged or irritated skin

Preparations & Dosing

Aloe can be applied topically to the skin as needed. It does not need to be rinsed off.

It is sometimes taken internally, but that is best undertaken with guidance from an herbalist or healthcare provider.

Contraindications

No contraindications for topical aloe.

Engels, G. (2010). Aloe. *HerbalGram*, (87), 1-5. http://cms.herbalgram.org/herbalgram/issue87/article3543.html.

Healthy Ingredients: Aloe. (n.d.). Retrieved from http://cms.herbalgram.org/healthyingredients/Aloe.html.

Levy, B. (1999). Re: Herbalist Reviews Literature on Aloe. *HerbClip Online*. http://cms.herbalgram.org/herbclip/161/review41934.html.

Apple Cider Vinegar

Apple cider vinegar is a simple kitchen remedy used for digestive, skin, and hair health.

Where to Buy

Apple cider vinegar is widely available in grocery stores and health food stores.

Buying Tips

The most effective apple cider vinegar for medicinal purposes is raw, unfiltered, and organic. This vinegar will contain a "mother," a naturally-occurring microbial colony.

Shelf Life

Apple cider vinegar is shelf-stable but use by the expiration date for best results.

Actions

- *Digestive*—improves digestive function
- *Balancing*—normalizes skin, scalp, and hair health

Preparations & Dosing

- Apple cider vinegar can be taken in water before or after meals, or on an empty stomach. One tablespoon mixed in water is an appropriate adult dose.
- It can be applied to the skin straight on small areas, or diluted in water over larger areas.
- One tablespoon in 1 cup of water can be used as a scalp and hair rinse.

Contraindications

Dental contact with straight apple cider vinegar can weaken tooth enamel over time. Always take diluted in water or mixed with food. When applied topically, straight apple cider vinegar may cause stinging or redness. Dilute with water as needed.

How to Make Your Own

Though apple cider vinegar can be brewed at home, it is a more advanced project.

Arnica

Arnica (*Arnica montana*) is a flowering herb used to treat bruises, sprains, and strains.

Where to Buy

Preparations can be found in large pharmacies or drugstores, health food stores, herbal shops, and Wellevate.

Buying Tips

Internal use of arnica is potentially toxic, but two formulations are safe. Homeopathic arnica is an extremely dilute preparation and comes in the form of small, white pellets that are taken under the tongue. Topical arnica uses the herbal or homeopathic extract in a lotion, cream, salve, or other topical preparation. Either version is acceptable, or you can keep both on hand.

Shelf Life

Most arnica preparations will be shelf-stable for approximately 1-3 years, but always check the individual product's expiration date.

Actions

- *Anti-inflammatory*—reduces pain, redness, and swelling associated with inflammation
- *Analgesic*—relieves pain
- *Vulnerary*—promotes healing of wounds and injuries

Preparations & Dosing

As stated above, arnica is best used topically and/or homeopathically. Follow package instructions for dosing homeopathic arnica.

Contraindications

Some individuals are allergic to arnica. If redness or itching develops after applying topical arnica, discontinue use. Do not use on broken or damaged skin.

How to Make Your Own

A simple arnica salve can be made by the following process:

1. Pour **4 ounces olive oil** over **¼ cup loosely packed dried arnica flowers** in a jar. Press the flowers down into the oil so all are covered, only adding more oil if needed. Cover the jar with a lid.
2. Place the jar in a small saucepan of water with a cloth at the bottom.
3. Set over very low heat for 3 hours, checking the pan occasionally to add more water if needed. The water should steam and can lightly simmer, but not boil hard.
4. Remove from heat and allow the oil to cool slightly, then pour through a cloth-lined sieve into a small, heat-safe jar or measuring cup.
5. Squeeze out as much oil as possible from the herb, then discard the herb.
6. Add **1 tablespoon beeswax pellets** to the herb-infused oil, then return to the saucepan of water.
7. Set over low heat again, bringing the water to simmer. Stir the oil and beeswax in the jar until the wax melts completely.
8. Remove the jar from the saucepan and allow the mixture to cool for a few minutes. Stir in up to 50 drops of quality **lavender essential oil** (optional) and pour into a 4-ounce tin or jar. Label with the product name, date created, and ingredients.

Arnica Flower (2000). *Expanded Commission E*. Retrieved from http://cms.herbalgram.org/expandedE/Arnicaflower.html.

Bone, K. & Mills, S. (2013). *Principles and Practice of Phytotherapy: Modern Herbal Medicine*. London: Elsevier.

Hoffmann, D. (2003). *Medical Herbalism: The Science and Practice of Herbal Medicine*. Rochester, VT: Healing Arts Press.

Baking Soda

Sodium bicarbonate, commonly known as baking soda, soothes itchy, irritated skin from bug bites and rashes.

Where to Buy

Baking soda can be found in the baking aisle of your grocery store.

Buying Tips

There's no need to buy special baking soda. The generic version at the store works just as well as name brands. It's also not necessary to buy baking soda labeled as "aluminum-free." It costs more and has been marketed due to confusion with baking *powder,* which often contains aluminum salts.

Shelf Life

Indefinitely, though it may start to take on odors of surrounding items if left in an opened box for extended lengths of time.

Actions

- *Anti-inflammatory*—soothes itching and redness from skin irritations

Preparations & Dosing

Baking soda can be mixed with water to create a paste that is applied to insect bites and stings. Allow the paste to dry, then remove and reapply if needed until the stinging is gone.

One cup of baking soda can also be added to a bath to calm rashes.

Contraindications

Baking soda pastes can be drying to the skin, so only use as needed.

Bentonite Clay

Bentonite clay is a grayish-tan clay that helps dry up rashes and acne.

Where to Buy

Bentonite clay can be found in health food stores and online retailers like Wellevate. Redmond Clay is a popular brand. (*Go to https://redmond.life/ collections/redmond-clay and use the code THRIVE at checkout to save 15%.*)

Buying Tips

Bentonite clay can be purchased as a dry powder or hydrated clay. Hydrated clay is more convenient, but dry powder is more economical.

Shelf Life

Dry clay will last indefinitely. Hydrated clay may come with an expiration date. The shelf-life can be extended by keeping the container sealed and away from additional moisture and contaminants.

Actions

- *Drying*—promotes healing of irritated skin conditions
- *Toning*—tones skin and tightens pores

Preparations & Dosage

Hydrated clay can be used as-is and smoothed over affected skin. Dry clay can be mixed with 1 part clay to 2 parts water and mixed with a non-metal utensil until a smooth paste forms.

Contraindications

Bentonite clay can be too drying for sensitive skin, so use with caution and rinse off before the clay paste can dry completely.

Carrier Oil

Any naturally cold- or expeller-pressed vegetable oil can work as a carrier oil. These are used to dilute essential oils, but they can also soothe dry skin and topical irritations on their own. Unrefined oils often have more skin-nourishing properties than those which have been deodorized or otherwise refined and processed.

Where to Buy

Some common carrier oils, like olive oil and coconut oil, are available at the grocery store with cooking oils. Specialty oils can be found at health food stores and online retailers that specialize in natural product formulation.

Buying Tips

There's no need to buy a fancy carrier oil unless you enjoy experimenting with uncommon options. Coconut and olive oils will likely be the most convenient and economical options, but some other choices are worth considering.

- Coconut oil is solid at room temperature and starts to melt at 76°F (25°C). Unrefined coconut oil smells like fresh coconuts, while refined versions have a neutral fragrance. It has a light feel and is quickly absorbed.
- Olive oil is heavy with a greasier feel than coconut oil. Extra virgin olive oil has a characteristic fragrance and yellowish-green hue, while refined olive oils have a lighter color and neutral scent.
- Grapeseed oil is very light on the skin and relatively neutral in fragrance. Because it has astringent action, it's a good choice for acne-prone skin.
- Sweet almond oil is a mild, neutral, nourishing oil for the skin. It's not greasy but feels heavier than coconut oil.
- Apricot kernel oil has similar properties to almond oil but is a better choice for those with nut allergies.
- Jojoba oil is technically a liquid wax. It's very similar to skin sebum and absorbs readily.

Shelf Life

Carrier oil shelf life varies depending on the specific oil and its level of refining. Most common carrier oils will last for a year or more. Exposure to light and high temperatures will cause carrier oils to go rancid more quickly.

Actions

Specific actions vary depending on the carrier oil. Most will be:

- *Emollient*—soothes skin
- *Vulnerary*—promotes wound healing

Many carrier oils, particularly unrefined carriers, can also help reduce skin inflammation.

Preparations & Dosage

Carrier oils can be applied topically as needed for dry skin, topical irritations, routine skincare, and diluting essential oils.

Contraindications

Generally none, but it is possible to be allergic to a carrier oil.

Parker, S. (2014). *Power of the Seed: Your Guide to Oils for Health and Beauty*. Port Townsend, WA: Process Media.

Cold & Flu Relief Tea

A simple blend of a few key herbs creates an effective remedy for common cold and flu symptoms like fever, congestion, and inflammation. Herbs often included in cold and flu formulas are yarrow (*Achillea millefolium*), elderflower (*Sambucus nigra*), peppermint (*Mentha piperita*), catnip (*Nepeta cataria*), chamomile (*Matricaria recutita*), ginger (*Zingiber officinalis*), and echinacea (*Echinacea* spp.).

Where to Buy

Many pharmacies and grocery stores now carry quality herbal teas. Health food stores will give you more options, as will online herbal retailers and herbalist-owned shops. My Wellevate protocol includes numerous Cold & Flu Relief Tea options.

Buying Tips

Herbal teas can be purchased in familiar boxes of tea bags or as loose herbal mixes. You can also purchase individual herbs separately and blend your own tea. Loose herbal tea allows you to easily see and smell the quality of herbs in the blend, though bagged herbal tea may seem more convenient. If you choose loose herbal tea, you'll need to purchase a few brewing tools like metal mesh tea strainers or reusable muslin tea bags.

Shelf Life

Dry herbal teas are best used within one year of purchase.

Actions

Specific actions vary depending on the specific herbs used in your herbal blend, but most will have the following actions:

- *Analgesic*—reduces pain levels
- *Anticatarrhal*—helps the body eliminate excess mucus and congestion
- *Antimicrobial*—helps the body rid itself of pathogenic microbes

- *Diaphoretic*—encourages sweating, which aids detoxification and regulates fever
- *Febrifuge*—moderates fever

Preparations & Dosage

Strong herbal teas are called infusions and can be made by steeping 1-2 teaspoons dried herb (or 1-2 teabags) in 1 cup of freshly boiled water for 30 minutes in a covered mug. Strain the herbs or remove the tea bags, then sweeten with honey if needed.

- Adults can take the tea 3-5 times daily during illness.
- Children ages 7-12 can take 2 cups of tea throughout the day.
- Children ages 2-6 can take 1 cup of tea throughout the day.

Contraindications

Most herbs in a cold and flu formula are safe, but yarrow (*Achillea millefolium*) and ginger (*Zingiber officinalis*) are contraindicated in medicinal doses during pregnancy.

How to Make Your Own

My favorite cold and flu herb blend contains **equal amounts of yarrow** (*Achillea millefolium*), **elderflower** (*Sambucus nigra*), and **peppermint** (*Mentha piperita*). These combine the most helpful herbal actions for cold and flu discomforts and it tastes great because of the mint. This blend is also kid-friendly, but not suitable for pregnancy.

1. Measure the herbs by weight (ideally) and place in a bowl to mix. A simple digital kitchen scale works great for measuring.
2. Combine the herbs completely, crushing any pieces that are substantially larger than the rest of the herb pieces.
3. Transfer to a glass jar and label with product name, herbs included, and blending date.

To use, follow the process above for brewing loose herbal infusions. During pregnancy, eliminate the yarrow.

Bone, K. & Mills, S. (2013). *Principles and Practice of Phytotherapy: Modern Herbal Medicine.* London: Elsevier.

Hoffmann, D. (2003). *Medical Herbalism: The Science and Practice of Herbal Medicine.* Rochester, VT: Healing Arts Press.

Echinacea Extract

Echinacea (*Echinacea* spp.) is a well-known flowering herb used for infections, particularly of the respiratory system. Both the root and the aerial parts are used medicinally in teas and extracts. I prefer keeping a combined extract of both the root and aerial parts in my medicine cabinet for quick and easy dosing, but any echinacea extract will do.

Where to Buy

Quality echinacea extracts are available in health food stores, online retailers, and small herbalist-owned shops. Two options are included in my Wellevate list.

Buying Tips

Alcohol-based extracts, called tinctures, are the standard extract type because alcohol can dissolve most of a plant's active compounds. The final product is also very shelf-stable. If you need to avoid alcohol, you can look for glycerites, extracts made with vegetable glycerine instead of alcohol. These are very sweet but free of sugar, making them kid-friendly.

A quality tincture or glycerite will be labeled with the species of echinacea (*E. purpurea*, *E. angustifolia*, or *E. pallida*) and plant part(s) used (root or herb). You should be able to see a ratio that describes how much plant material was used in the solvent. Echinacea tinctures and glycerites are often a 1:5 extract, meaning 1 gram of herb is extracted in every 5 milliliters of liquid.

Shelf Life

Theoretically, tinctures will last indefinitely, but they are best used within 3-5 years.

Actions

- *Alterative*—supports natural detoxification through the lymphatic system
- *Anti-inflammatory*—reduces pain, redness, and swelling from inflammation
- *Antimicrobial*—boosts the body's efforts to fight off pathogenic microbes
- *Immunomodulator*—encourages healthy immune response

Preparations & Dosage

Echinacea extract can be taken straight from the dropper or added to a small amount of water or juice. Dosing will vary depending on the extract's strength, so follow dosing guidelines on the package.

Contraindications

Echinacea may cause allergic reactions to people sensitive to the daisy (Asteraceae) family. It is likely safe during pregnancy when used for a short time, such as during an infection. It is not suitable for individuals on immunosuppressant therapies.

How to Make Your Own

Though tinctures seem intimidating, they only require some special ingredients and a kitchen scale. You can make a 1:5 echinacea tincture like this:

1. Take **20 grams dried echinacea herb** and **20 grams dried echinacea root** and pulse in a clean coffee grinder until the herb is in small, uniform pieces. It doesn't need to be powdered, but the pieces should be very small.
2. Place the ground herb in a clean glass jar and add **200 milliliters of 100-proof vodka** (or other neutral alcohol). Conversely, add 140 milliliters vegetable glycerine and 60 milliliters water for an alcohol-free extract.
3. Cap the jar and shake to fully disperse the herb through the vodka, then place in a cabinet.

4. Shake the jar daily (or as often as you remember) for around 3 weeks.
5. Strain the liquid through a cloth-lined sieve. Thin kitchen towels or double layers of cheesecloth work well for this. Squeeze out as much liquid as possible to get all the tincture you can.
6. Pour the tincture into a 4-ounce dark amber glass bottle, then cap and label with the extract name, date made, and ingredients.

Adults can take ½ teaspoon (or 2.5 milliliters) 3-5 times daily during sickness.

For children, take their approximate weight in pounds and divide it by 150. This gives you the fraction of an adult dose that is suitable for them.

For example, a 50-pound child would get 50/150 (or ⅓) of an adult dose. There are approximately 100 drops in a teaspoon, making 50 drops a single adult dose. One-third of 50 is about 17, making 17 drops of tincture a suitable dose for a 50-pound child.

Bone, K. & Mills, S. (2013). *Principles and Practice of Phytotherapy: Modern Herbal Medicine.* London: Elsevier.

Echinacea Purpurea Herb. (2000). *Expanded Commission E.* Retrieved from http://cms.herbalgram.org/expandedE/EchinaceaPurpureaherb.html.

Echinacea Purpurea Root. (2000). *Expanded Commission E.* Retrieved from http://cms.herbalgram.org/expandedE/EchinaceaPurpurearoot.html.

Hoffmann, D. (2003). *Medical Herbalism: The Science and Practice of Herbal Medicine.* Rochester, VT: Healing Arts Press.

Elderberry Syrup or Gummies

Elderberry (*Sambucus nigra*) is a wonderful herb that boosts immunity and helps shorten the duration of colds and flu. It is best prepared by cooking, so syrups or gummies are an easy way to take the herb.

Where to Buy

Elderberry syrup and gummies are becoming widely available in many supermarkets and pharmacies. You can also find elderberry preparations at health food stores, online retailers like Wellevate, and small herbalist-owned shops.

Buying Tips

- Sugar or honey is required to make syrup, but pay attention to the amount included, especially with gummies.
- Store-bought syrups will include a preservative. I prefer a small amount of alcohol as a preservative over other options.
- Small-batch, herbalist-made syrups may be completely free of preservatives.
- Gummies may include extra flavorings, gums, and waxes, so read labels carefully.

Shelf Life

Elderberry syrup made without additional preservatives and homemade elderberry gummies will keep 2-4 weeks in the refrigerator. Store-bought versions may last longer, but check the expiration dates to be sure.

Actions

- *Antiviral*—binds viruses and inhibits viral replication; protects against viral infection
- *Diaphoretic*—promotes sweating when taken at sufficient doses
- *Immunostimulant*—strengthens immune function

Preparations & Dosage

Elderberry is best taken as a cooked preparation. It contains a compound in the seeds (hydrocyanic acid) that can cause nausea and vomiting in some sensitive people. Elderberry syrup and gummies are both cooked preparations.

Since elderberry is also a food, dosing is very flexible. Suggested dosing might be:

- Adults can take up to 1 tablespoon daily to protect against infection, or 1 tablespoon 3-5 times a day when sick.
- Older children can take 2 teaspoons daily as a preventative, or 2 teaspoons 3-5 times a day during sickness.
- Young children can take 1 teaspoon daily as a preventative, or 1 teaspoon 3-5 times a day when sick.

Contraindications

None known

How to Make Your Own

Elderberry syrup is very easy to make.

1. Take **100 grams dried elderberries** (about 1 cup) and place them in a saucepan with **4 cups cold water**. Allow to soak for 30-60 minutes, if possible.
2. Bring the water to a gentle boil and continue boiling until the water is reduced by half. This will take another 30-60 minutes.
3. Strain out the liquid (now called a decoction) through a fine-mesh sieve. Press the cooked berries with the back of a spoon to press out any remaining liquid. You should have 2 cups of elderberry decoction. If you don't have enough, return the berries to the pan and cook with more water to make 2 cups. If you have too much, return the decoction to the pan without the berries and cook off some of the extra water.

4. For a simple syrup, allow the decoction to cool, then add **1-2 cups local, raw honey** and stir to combine. This syrup will be very thin, but it will contain the benefits of raw honey, as well. More honey will result in a longer shelf life. Store in the refrigerator and use within 2 (for 1 cup honey) or 4 (for 2 cups honey) weeks.

5. For a thicker syrup, add **1 ½ cups cane sugar** instead of honey to the elderberry decoction in a pan. Boil again until the mixture thickens into a syrup. Store in the refrigerator and use within 4 weeks.

Dose as suggested above.

Buhner, S. H. (2013). *Herbal Antivirals: Natural Remedies for Emerging & Resistant Viral Infections*. North Adams, MA: Storey Publishing.

Garner-Wizard, M. (2006). Re: Review of Pharmacology and Clinical Benefits of European Elderberry. *HerbClip*. Retrieved from http://cms.herbalgram.org/herbclip/297/review44356.html.

Hoffmann, D. (2003). *Medical Herbalism: The Science and Practice of Herbal Medicine*. Rochester, VT: Healing Arts Press.

Epsom Salt

Epsom salt isn't actually salt at all. It's magnesium sulfate, but its whitish-clear, granular appearance looks like salt. It offers a simple way to boost magnesium levels, soothe sore or injured muscles and joints, and promote restful sleep.

Where to Buy

Epsom salt is widely available at pharmacies, supermarkets, and big-box stores.

Buying Tips

You can find Epsom salt in 2-pound cartons and bags of many sizes. Avoid scented Epsom salts as these usually contain artificial fragrances.

Shelf Life

Epsom salt will last indefinitely, but it may clump if it's exposed to moisture over time.

Actions

- *Mineral supplement*—boosts magnesium levels
- *Vulnerary*—helps injuries heal

Preparations & Dosage

Epsom salt can be used in a bath, either local (like a foot soak) or whole body.

- Add ½-1 cup of Epsom salt to a large bowl or basin and fill with warm water for a localized soak.
- Add 2 cups of Epsom salt to the bathtub for a full bath. Soak for 20-30 minutes.

Contraindications

None

Essential Oils

Essential oils are highly concentrated plant extracts made of a plant's volatile oil. Some people rely on them entirely for their natural medicine cabinet, while others find them so intimidating they avoid them completely. The best approach is somewhere in the middle.

Essential oils are a valuable addition to your Minimalist Natural Medicine Cabinet, but that doesn't mean you need a large, expensive set of oils. One to five carefully chosen essential oils will cover most household needs.

Where to Buy

Essential oils are becoming easier to find every day. Most health food stores and even some pharmacies carry them, but the best selection is most easily found online through various retailers. Some are listed in my Wellevate list, but you can find more options on the Recommended Products page on my website: https://abetterwaytothrive.com/recommended-products.

Buying Tips

There are many quality essential oil brands. Look for brands that:

- Provide batch-specific GC/MS test reports.
- Sell certified organic or sustainably wildcrafted essential oils.
- Label their essential oils with the common name, botanical name, and country of origin.
- Sell their essential oils at various price points, depending on the source plant material.
- Provide safe, evidence-based information free of hype and reckless claims.

Terms like "therapeutic grade," "100% pure," and "all natural" are marketing terms without concrete meanings. If a brand uses any of these to describe their essential oils, you can contact them and ask them what they mean.

Shelf Life

Essential oil shelf life varies depending on the specific oil. Citrus oils have the shortest shelf life and can start to oxidize after just 6 months. Other oils can last for many years.

For best results with most essential oils, store them in a cool, dark cabinet that retains a consistent temperature and only buy as much as you can use within 12 months.

Actions

Specific actions are shared under each individual essential oil.

Preparations & Dosage

Specific preparations are shared under each individual essential oil, but some safety guidelines are universal.

- Always dilute essential oils in a carrier oil when applying topically. Neat, meaning undiluted, essential oil application can lead to irritation, sensitivity reactions, and even allergic reactions after repeated exposure.
- Essential oils should only be used internally with the guidance and oversight of a certified aromatherapist with training in aromatic medicine, along with cooperation from your licensed healthcare provider.
- Never drink essential oils added to water.
- Use caution when diffusing around animals, infants, young children, pregnant women, the elderly, and anyone whose health history you are unfamiliar with. Light diffusion of mild essential oils in a large room is generally safe, but courteous caution is still warranted.
- Avoid contact with eyes, mucous membranes, and other sensitive tissue.

General dilution guidelines are as follows:

- For infants up to 2 years old, a .25% dilution of lavender (*Lavandula angustifolia*) is suitable in a baby massage oil. This is approximately 1 drop essential oil in 4 teaspoons carrier oil.
- For children ages 2-6, a .5% dilution of lavender and other mild essential oils is suitable for whole-body use (1 drop in 2 teaspoons carrier), or 1-2% for localized treatments (1-2 drops per teaspoon carrier).
- For children ages 7-12, a 1% dilution of safe essential oils is suitable for whole-body use (1 drop in 1 teaspoons carrier), or 2-5% for localized treatments (2-5 drops per teaspoon carrier).
- For adults, a 1-2% dilution is suitable for whole-body applications (1-2 drops per teaspoon carrier), or 3-10% for localized treatments (3-10 drops per teaspoon carrier).

For thorough dilution guidelines, including printable charts for infants, children, adults, pregnant women, and elderly adults, please see my printable resource *The Essential Oils Quick Reference Guide*.

To get a strong foundation with essential oils, see my book *Essential Oils: Separation Truth from Myth*, available in print, PDF, and Kindle.

Both resources can be found here: https://abetterwaytothrive.com/shop.

Contraindications

Specific contraindications are listed below for each individual essential oil.

Specific Essential Oils to Include

The following essential oils are excellent additions to your Minimalist Natural Medicine Cabinet. You don't need to buy all of them if you find that intimidating or cost-prohibitive. I've listed them according to importance, but use the descriptions to help you decide which ones you want to include if you need to choose some over others.

Lavender (Lavandula angustifolia)

If you only want to add one essential oil to your natural medicine cabinet, choose lavender. It's been used for hundreds of years, demonstrating its safety and versatility. There are a few species of lavender essential oil, so look for the botanical names *Lavandula angustifolia*, *L. vera*, or *L. officinalis/ officinale* which are all synonyms for the same plant.

Actions

- *Analgesic*—reduces pain
- *Anti-inflammatory*—reduces pain, redness, and swelling from inflammation
- *Antimicrobial*—reduces pathogenic microbes
- *Antispasmodic*—reduces muscle spasms, cramps, and tension
- *Nervine Tonic*—promotes a balanced nervous system
- *Vulnerary*—promotes wound healing

Preparations & Dosage

Lavender is useful for burns, bug bites, rashes, headaches, restlessness, stress, and more.

- A drop can be placed on a cotton ball or tissue for inhalation.
- It can be diluted in a carrier oil and applied topically.
- It can be added to a diffuser for inhalation.
- Five drops can be mixed with 1 teaspoon *each* carrier oil and liquid soap, then added to bathwater.

Lavender is one of the gentlest oils, useful for the whole family.

Contraindications

None.

Sweet Orange (Citrus sinensis)

Sweet orange is one of my favorite citrus essential oils. It has a lovely aroma and offers various benefits. And while many citrus essential oils will cause phototoxicity, a painful reaction from exposure to sunlight after topical application, sweet orange will not.

Actions

- *Antidepressant*—boosts mood
- *Antiemetic*—reduces nausea
- *Carminative*—reduces intestinal gas and bloating
- *Digestive*—boosts digestive function
- *Nervine Relaxant*—promotes a calm central nervous system

Preparations & Dosage

Sweet orange essential oil is a helpful essential oil for nerve-related needs. It can promote restful sleep while boosting mood at the same time.

- A drop can be placed on a cotton ball or tissue for inhalation.
- It can be mixed with a carrier and applied topically.
- It can be added to a diffuser for inhalation.
- It can be added to homemade cleaning sprays.

Lavender and sweet orange make a wonderful, balancing blend that can promote calm focus and relaxation. This combination is especially suited for sensitive individuals like children, pregnant women, and the elderly.

Contraindications

None, though strong topical dilutions can cause unpleasant burning or tingling sensations on the skin.

Eucalyptus (Eucalyptus globulus, E. radiata, or E. smithii)

There have been some fearful reports claiming eucalyptus is a dangerous essential oil for children, making some parents afraid to keep it around. But it offers too many benefits to skip, especially when it can be used safely.

Actions

- *Analgesic*—reduces pain
- *Antimicrobial*—reduces pathogenic microbes
- *Antiseptic*—helps protect against infections
- *Decongestant*—reduces mucus congestion in the respiratory system
- *Expectorant*—thins and loosens mucus so it can be expelled
- *Rubefacent*—increases circulation to a localized area of the body

Preparations & Dosage

Eucalyptus can be used topically and through inhalation. It's most widely used for respiratory support.

- It can be mixed with a carrier oil at appropriate dilutions and applied to the chest as a decongestant and expectorant.
- It can be diluted and applied topically over painful areas.
- It can be used in homemade cleaning sprays.
- A drop can be placed on a cotton ball or tissue for inhalation.
- It can be used in a diffuser for inhalation.

Eucalyptus blends well with lavender as a respiratory support for children. Eucalyptus and peppermint (mentioned below) can be combined for adult respiratory support.

Contraindications

Eucalyptus essential oil is best avoided by children under 2 years old.

For children ages 2-10, *Eucalyptus radiata* or *E. smithii* are safer species than *E. globulus*. They contain less 1,8-cineole, also known as eucalyptol. This chemical can be toxic in high doses for young children.

For children ages 12 and up, as well as adults, any eucalyptus species is suitable.

Tea Tree (Melaleuca alternifolia)

Tea tree is a highly effective oil for wound care and disinfecting. It's a helpful addition to skin salves, spot treatments for acne, and homemade cleaning sprays.

Actions

- *Anti-inflammatory*—reduces pain, redness, and swelling from inflammation
- *Antimicrobial*—reduces pathogenic microbes, including viruses, bacteria, and fungi
- *Antiseptic*—helps protect against infection
- *Immunostimulant*—boosts immune response
- *Vulnerary*—promotes wound healing

Preparations & Dosage

Tea tree oil has a very medicinal aroma, making it best suited for topical use and cleaning purposes.

- It can be added to healing salves at appropriate dilutions.
- It can be diluted in a carrier oil and applied to cuts, scrapes, bruises, bug bites, pimples, rashes, and other skin irritations.
- It can be added to homemade cleaning sprays for antimicrobial purposes.

Contraindications

None.

Peppermint (Mentha piperita)

Peppermint is an energizing oil that also helps with pain. It's strong and demands a careful approach, but it's very useful and worth having available.

Actions

- *Analgesic*—reduces pain
- *Antispasmodic*—reduces muscle cramps, spasms, and tension
- *Carminative*—reduces intestinal gas and bloating
- *Decongestant*—reduces mucus congestion of the respiratory system
- *Expectorant*—thins and loosens mucus so it can be expelled
- *Febrifuge*—regulates fever
- *Rubefacient*—increases localized circulation

Preparations & Dosage

Peppermint is well-suited for inhalation and careful topical application.

- A drop can be placed on a cotton ball or tissue for inhalation.
- It can be diluted in a carrier oil and applied topically over localized areas.

Contraindications

Peppermint is best avoided by children under 6 and used carefully with children under 10. Spearmint (*Mentha spicata*) is a gentler option for children.

Peppermint requires milder dilutions to avoid unpleasant skin reactions.

Keville, K. & Green, M. (2009). *Aromatherapy: A Complete Guide to the Healing Art* (2nd ed.). Berkeley, CA: Crossing Press.

Lawless, J. (2014). *The Encyclopedia of Essential Oils: The Complete Guide to the Use of Aromatic Oils in Aromatherapy, Herbalism, Health, and Well-Being.* New York, NY: Falls River Press.

Price, S. & Price, P. (2012). *Aromatherapy for Health Professionals* (4th ed.). London: Elsevier.

Rhind, J. P. (2012). *Essential Oils: A Handbook for Aromatherapy Practice* (2nd ed.). London: Singing Dragon.

Garlic

Garlic (*Allium sativum*) is a useful all-purpose antimicrobial you can find at any grocery store. It can help protect against illness and encourage a healthy immune response when sickness does occur.

Where to Buy

Almost all grocery stores carry garlic. Health food stores, local food co-ops, and farm markets are more likely to carry local and/or organically grown garlic.

Buying Tips

Look for garlic bulbs that are firm and show no signs of greening or sprouting at the tips of each clove. Ideally, purchase garlic grown in the USA (or your home country). Minced, jarred garlic is fine for culinary use, but won't be as medicinally useful as fresh garlic.

Shelf Life

Fresh garlic bulbs will last 6-12 months, depending on the time of harvest, type of garlic, country of origin, and other factors. Store it in a cool, dry place as you would onions and potatoes.

Actions

- *Antimicrobial*—boosts the body's efforts to fight off pathogenic microbes
- *Antispasmodic*—reduces muscle spasms, cramps, and tension
- *Diaphoretic*—encourages sweating to aid detoxification and regulate fever
- *Expectorant*—thins and loosens mucus congestion so it can be expelled
- *Hypotensive*—promotes a lowered, healthy blood pressure when blood pressure is elevated

Preparations & Dosage

Garlic can be used fresh, cooked, or in capsules.

- Fresh garlic can be sprinkled on foods just before consuming or taken in a spoonful of honey (honey is especially helpful for children).
- To retain the medicinal properties of garlic when cooking, finely mince it, allow it to set out exposed to air for about 10 minutes, and then add to the recipe.
- Garlic capsules are available as powder capsules, extract capsules, and aged garlic extract capsules. These may be easier to take if you don't like the taste or smell of garlic, but they require a specialized purchase.

As a food, dosing for garlic is flexible. Suggested dosing may be:

- For adults, one clove fresh garlic can be taken daily for immune support. During sickness, the dose can be increased to 3-5 times per day.
- Children ages 7-12 can take 2 cloves total finely minced garlic throughout the day, either added to food or taken with honey during sickness.
- Children ages 2-6, 1 clove total finely minced garlic can be given throughout the day, either added to food or taken with honey during sickness.

Contraindications

High therapeutic doses of garlic should be avoided by anyone on blood-thinning medications and ceased 2 weeks before surgical procedures.

High doses of garlic, especially fresh, may cause nausea. Reduce the dose or cease taking it if nausea occurs.

How to Grow Your Own

Garlic is a fun, carefree plant to grow if you have a little yard space. It is typically planted in the fall, allowed to overwinter, and then starts growing in the spring.

In the spring, thick, curly, edible stems called scapes come up. These are cut off to encourage healthy bulb formation and are simply delicious! Once the leaves start to die back in the late summer or early fall, the garlic can be pulled, cured, and stored to enjoy until the next season.

Reach out to a local garden club, visit an organic gardening website, or check out a gardening book from the library for more information on growing garlic.

Fritchey, P. (2004). *Practical Herbalism: Ordinary Plants with Extraordinary Powers*. Warsaw, IN: Whitman Publications.

Garlic. (1988). *Commission E Monographs*. Retrieved from http://cms.herbalgram.org/commissione/Monographs/Monograph0179.html.

Garlic. (2000). *Expanded Commission E*. Retrieved from http://cms.herbalgram.org/expandedE/Garlic.html.

Hoffmann, D. (2003). *Medical Herbalism: The Science and Practice of Herbal Medicine*. Rochester, VT: Healing Arts Press.

Ginger

Ginger (*Zingiber officinale*) is another natural medicine cabinet staple easily found in most grocery stores. It's beneficial for stomach, respiratory, and circulatory concerns.

Where to Buy

Ginger root (technically a rhizome) is widely available in large grocery stores and health food stores in the refrigerated produce section. Dry and powdered ginger is found in the spice aisle, but it is often not as potent as the fresh root. Pre-made extracts, capsules, and teas can be found in health food stores, large pharmacies, and online retailers.

Buying Tips

Look for firm ginger with smooth skin and avoid any that appear wrinkled or feel spongy.

Shelf Life

Ginger can last up to a month in the refrigerator. Once cut, place in a sealed container, beeswax wrap, or plastic bag to prevent moisture loss.

Actions

- *Antiemetic*—reduces nausea and helps prevent vomiting
- *Anti-inflammatory*—reduces pain, swelling, and redness from inflammation
- *Antispasmodic*—reduces muscle cramps, spasms, and tension
- *Carminative*—reduces intestinal gas and bloating
- *Diaphoretic*—encourages sweating to promote natural detoxification and regulate fever
- *Digestive*—stimulates healthy digestive function
- *Rubefacient*—promotes circulation to a specific area when applied topically

Preparations & Dosage

Like garlic, ginger can be used liberally in the diet. Common medicinal preparations include:

- For an infusion, slice a 1-inch piece of washed ginger and place in the bottom of a mug. Pour 1 cup of freshly boiled water over it, then cover and steep for 30 minutes. More hot water can be added until the ginger loses its flavor.
- For a decoction, add 4 1-inch pieces of washed ginger to 4 cups of water in a small saucepan. Cover the pan, bring to a boil, then reduce heat to a simmer. Continue simmering gently for 30 minutes, checking regularly to add more water if needed. Allow to cool and drink throughout the day.
- Finely shred or mince a small piece of ginger, then combine with enough honey to make a thin paste. Spread on toast or use in teas. Store in the refrigerator.
- Finely shred ginger and place in a heat-safe bowl. Pour over enough freshly boiled water to cover the ginger, then allow to steep while covered. Once cool, soak a cloth in the strong infusion and apply topically as a compress. The shredded ginger can also be folded inside the cloth and applied topically as a poultice.

Like elderberry and garlic, dosing for ginger is flexible. Suggested dosing may be:

- For adults, 1 cup infusion or decoction can be taken every 2-3 hours, or throughout the day as needed.
- For children ages 7-12, 2 cups total infusion or decoction can be taken daily.
- For children ages 2-6, 1 cup total infusion or decoction can be taken daily.
- For compresses and poultices, leave on the skin for 20-30 minutes, or until the area is warmed and pain is relieved.

Contraindications

Strong doses of ginger can cause a warming sensation in the stomach. If this becomes unpleasant or turns into nausea, reduce the dose or cease taking it.

In some herbal texts, ginger is contraindicated in pregnancy because it is sometimes classified as an emmenagogue (a substance that promotes menstruation). However, ginger is regularly used in some herbal traditions as a morning sickness remedy. Until more is understood, ginger should be used with caution at therapeutic doses during pregnancy, especially by women with a history of miscarriage. Culinary use of ginger during pregnancy is safe.

Bone, K. & Mills, S. (2013). *Principles and Practice of Phytotherapy: Modern Herbal Medicine*. London: Elsevier.

Comments on Specific Monographs. (n.d.) *The Commission E Monographs*. Retrieved from http://cms.herbalgram.org/commissione/ednotes.html.

Ginger Root. (2000). *Herbal Medicine: Expanded Commission E*. Retrieved from http://cms.herbalgram.org/expandedE/Gingerroot.html.

Ginger Root. (1988). *The Commission E Monographs*. Retrieved from http://cms.herbalgram.org/commissione/Monographs/Monograph0181.html.

Hoffmann, D. (2003). *Medical Herbalism: The Science and Practice of Herbal Medicine*. Rochester, VT: Healing Arts Press.

Healing Salve

A good herbal healing salve is made from herb-infused oils, like olive or coconut, thickened with beeswax, and often boosted with skin-loving essential oils. Common herbs used in healing salves are chickweed (*Stellaria media*), plantain leaf (*Plantago major*), calendula (*Calendula officinalis*), comfrey (*Symphytum officinale*), echinacea (*Echinacea* spp.), lavender (*Lavandula angustifolia*), St. John's wort (*Hypericum perforatum*), and others. It's helpful for almost all skin complaints.

Where to Buy

Herbal healing salves are available in some large pharmacies, health food stores, large online retailers like Wellevate, and herbalist-owned shops.

Buying Tips

Look for salves free of petroleum ingredients, like mineral oil or petroleum jelly. Herbs should be listed with their common and botanical names.

Preservatives aren't needed in salves, so avoid any that use them. The exception may be if a salve was made from fresh herbs. Fresh herbs introduce water into the final product and shorten the shelf life, sometimes substantially. I prefer salves made from properly dried herbs.

If essential oils are included, look for gentle additions like lavender (*Lavandula angustifolia*) and tea tree (*Melaleuca alternifolia*), but avoid salves that contain potentially irritating oils like oregano (*Origanum vulgare*).

Shelf Life

Salves are best used within a year but can be used longer if they show no signs of spoilage. To encourage a long shelf life, use care when taking the salve out of a container and avoid introducing dirt, microbes, and other contaminants.

Actions

Actions will vary depending on the specific herbs used in your salve, but most will have the following actions:

- *Analgesic*—reduces pain
- *Anti-inflammatory*—reduces pain, redness, and swelling from inflammation
- *Antimicrobial*—helps the body resist pathogenic microbes
- *Astringent*—tones and tightens tissue
- *Emollient*—soothes irritated skin
- *Vulnerary*—promotes wound healing

Preparations & Dosage

Healing salves can be used as needed and applied directly over cuts, scrapes, bruises, rashes, insect bites, and other irritations. There's no need to rinse off.

Contraindications

None, though long-term exposure to high doses of comfrey (*Symphytum officinale*) on broken or damaged skin is best avoided.

Some herbs encourage skin regeneration so profoundly that they may cause the skin to grow together over a deep cut before the lower tissue has had time to heal. Seek medical care for deep cuts and wounds which require stitches.

How to Make Your Own

I've been making the following salve recipe for years. It's a mainstay in our home and a go-to gift for my family at Christmas. I've heard wonderful reports from everyone who uses it, including soothing eczema, reducing scars, and speeding incision healing after surgery.

6. Take **1/2 cup packed herbs** and place in a glass pint jar. My favorite combination is **equal parts chickweed** (*Stellaria media*), **calendula** (*Calendula officinalis*), and **plantain** (*Plantago major*), but you can simply use just one of them.
7. Pour **1 cup carrier oil** over the herbs (I often use equal parts olive oil and coconut oil). Add a cap to the jar.
8. Place the jar in a small saucepan of water with a cloth at the bottom.
9. Set over very low heat for 3 hours, checking the pan occasionally to add more water if needed. The water should steam or lightly simmer, but not boil hard.
10. Remove from heat and allow the oil to cool slightly, then pour the oil through a cloth-lined sieve into a small heat-safe jar or measuring cup.
11. Squeeze out as much oil as possible from the herb, then discard the herb.
12. Add **2 tablespoons beeswax pellets** to the herb-infused oil, then return to the saucepan of water with the cloth at the bottom.
13. Set over low heat again, bringing the water to simmer. Stir the oil and beeswax in the jar until the wax melts completely.
14. Remove the jar from the saucepan and allow the mixture to cool for a few minutes. Stir in up to 50 drops *each* quality **lavender and tea tree essential oil** (optional) and pour into two 4-ounce tins or jars. Label with the name, date created, and ingredients.

Both chickweed and plantain are common weeds that grow abundantly in unsprayed yards. Look for chickweed in the early spring and fall. Plantain grows best in the early summer and early fall. Calendula is an easy garden plant that can be grown in containers.

Fritchey, P. (2004). *Practical Herbalism: Ordinary Plants with Extraordinary Powers*. Warsaw, IN: Whitman Publications.

Hoffmann, D. (2003). *Medical Herbalism: The Science and Practice of Herbal Medicine*. Rochester, VT: Healing Arts Press.

Honey

Honey isn't just used to sweeten your tea. It's an amazing remedy on its own! For your natural medicine cabinet, local, raw wildflower honey is ideal.

Where to Buy

Most large grocery stores will carry good, locally-produced honey. Health food stores will likely offer a better selection. Farm markets may be the best source.

Buying Tips

Look for honey that is raw and lightly filtered. It may look a little cloudy, which likely means it contains some pollen and/or propolis. Honey sourced from just one plant, like clover or alfalfa, won't offer the same medicinal benefits as wildflower honey. Specialty manuka honey is much more expensive than local wildflower honey and not necessary as a natural home remedy.

Shelf Life

Honey lasts indefinitely.

Actions

- *Antiallergenic*—reduces allergy symptoms and allergy response
- *Anti-inflammatory*—reduces pain, redness, and swelling from inflammation
- *Antimicrobial*—reduces pathogenic microbes
- *Antioxidant*—reduces harmful oxidation processes
- *Immunostimulant*—encourages healthy and robust immune response
- *Expectorant*—thins and loosens mucus so it can be expelled
- *Vulnerary*—promotes wound healing

Preparations & Dosage

Honey can be used both topically and internally for many purposes:

- It can be added to herbal infusions and decoctions to sweeten and add medicinal benefits.
- It can be taken straight for cough relief and immune support.
- It can be applied topically to burns and cuts, then covered with a clean bandage, to promote healing.
- It can be used as a face mask for acne, or simply to promote skin health.

As a food product, dosing for honey is flexible. Suggested dosing may be:

- Adults can take 1 tablespoon of honey as needed throughout the day during acute situations like coughs, colds, flu, and allergies.
- Children ages 1-10 can take as adults, using 1-2 teaspoons per dose throughout the day.

As mentioned previously, honey can also be combined with fresh garlic and/or ginger to combat infection and promote recovery during an illness.

Contraindications

Honey is not safe for infants under 1 year.

Buhner, S. H. (2012). *Herbal Antibiotic: Natural Alternatives for Drug-Resistant Bacteria*. North Adams, MA: Storey Publishing.

Oppel, M. N. (2008). *Re: Study Finds Honey More Effective than Dexromethorphan for Children's Nighttime Cough*. HerbClip. Retrieved from http://cms.herbalgram.org/herbclip/358/review020688-358.html.

Re: Review of Bee Products: Honey, Pollen, Propolis, and Royal Jelly. (1999). HerbClip. Retrieved from http://cms.herbalgram.org/herbclip/166/review42360.html.

Lemon

Lemons, with their tart juice and comforting, cheerful aroma, can help alleviate many uncomfortable symptoms and help other remedies go down easier.

Where to Buy

Fresh lemons can be found at almost all grocery stores.

Buying Tips

If you plan to use the lemon zest, or yellow outer peel, be sure to purchase organic lemons. Conventional lemons are fine if you will only use the juice, can't find organic lemons, and/or find organic options cost-prohibitive.

Shelf Life

Lemons will last around 2 weeks in the refrigerator.

Actions

- *Anti-inflammatory*—reduces pain, redness, and swelling from inflammation
- *Antioxidant*—reduces harmful oxidation processes
- *Astringent*—tones and tightens tissue
- *Nutrient*—provides needed nutrients, particularly Vitamin C

Preparations & Dosage

Freshly squeezed lemon juice can be liberally used in the diet, added to herbal infusions and decoctions, and added to honey for a quick cough remedy.

A quick rehydration drink can be made with the freshly squeezed juice from half a lemon, a teaspoon of honey, and a pinch of sea salt mixed into a cup of water.

Contraindications

None.

Lemon. (n.d.) *Healthy Ingredients*. Retrieved from
http://cms.herbalgram.org/healthyingredients/Lemon.html.

Relaxing Nervine Tea

Relaxant nervines are herbs that promote a calm nervous system. A blend of relaxant nervine herbs is helpful during times of stress, occasional anxiety, difficulty sleeping, and similar concerns. Chamomile (*Matricaria recutita*), lemon balm (*Melissa officinalis*), lavender (*Lavandula angustifolia*), catnip (*Nepeta cataria*), linden (*Tilia platyphyllos*), skullcap (*Scutellaria lateriflora*), and passionflower (*Passiflora incarnata*) are common relaxant nervines that can be used alone or in combination.

Where to Buy

Many pharmacies and grocery stores now carry quality herbal teas. Health food stores will give you more options, as will online herbal retailers and herbalist-owned online shops. My Wellevate list includes numerous Relaxing Nervine Tea options.

Buying Tips

Herbal teas can be purchased in familiar boxes of tea bags or as loose herbal mixes. You can also purchase individual herbs separately and blend your own tea. Loose herbal tea allows you to easily see and smell the quality of herbs in the blend, though bagged herbal tea may seem more convenient. If you choose loose herbal tea, you'll need to purchase a few brewing tools like metal mesh tea strainers or reusable muslin tea bags.

Shelf Life

Dry herbal teas are best used within one year of purchase.

Actions

Specific actions will vary depending on the individual herbs in your blend, but most will have the following actions:

- *Antispasmodic*—reduces muscle spasms, cramps, and tension
- *Carminative*—relieves intestinal gas and bloating
- *Relaxant Nervine*—calms the nervous system

Preparations & Dosage

Strong herbal teas are called infusions and can be made by steeping 1-2 teaspoons dried herb (or 1-2 teabags) in 1 cup of freshly boiled water for 30 minutes in a covered mug. Strain the herbs or remove the tea bags if you'd like, then sweeten with honey if desired.

Because the herbs in relaxant nervine teas tend to be very gentle, dosing is flexible.

- Adults can take the tea 3-5 times daily during periods of stress, or once daily as part of an evening routine.
- Children ages 7-12 can take 1 cup as needed.
- Children ages 2-6 can take ½ cup of tea as needed.

Contraindications

Most relaxant nervine herbs are generally safe. Passionflower (*Passiflora incarnata*) is a sedative herb with a stronger relaxant action, so choosing milder relaxants, such as chamomile (*Matricaria recutita*) and lemon balm (*Melissa officinalis*), can be a wise choice for young children.

Passionflower may increase the effectiveness of over-the-counter or pre-scription sedatives.

How to Make Your Own

A simple chamomile infusion is the classic relaxant tea. It has a comforting flavor, is safe for all ages, as well as during pregnancy and lactation, and is effective on its own.

As an herbalist, though, I can't help but blend it with two other gentle, relaxing herbs. I love combining **equal amounts of chamomile** (*Matricaria recutita*), **lemon balm** (*Melissa officinalis*), and **catnip** (*Nepeta cataria*) for a lovely, restful tea. It's best if you can measure these by weight, but measuring by volume works in a pinch for this combination.

1. Measure the herbs and place in a bowl to mix.
2. Combine the herbs completely, crushing any pieces that are substantially larger than the rest of the herb pieces.
3. Transfer to a glass jar and label with name, herbs included, and blending date.

To use, follow the process above for brewing loose herbal infusions.

Bone, K. & Mills, S. (2013). *Principles and Practice of Phytotherapy: Modern Herbal Medicine*. London: Elsevier.

Fritchey, P. (2004). *Practical Herbalism: Ordinary Plants with Extraordinary Powers*. Warsaw, IN: Whitman Publications.

Hoffmann, D. (2003). *Medical Herbalism: The Science and Practice of Herbal Medicine*. Rochester, VT: Healing Arts Press.

Romm, A. (2018). *Botanical Medicine for Women's Health* (2nd ed.). St. Louis, MO: Elsevier.

Sea Salt

Simple sea salt can be used with water and oil for several remedies, including washes, baths, scrubs, gargles, and more.

Where to Buy

Sea salt is available in most grocery stores, in health food stores, and through online retailers. Real Salt from Redmond is what I personally use and recommend most often. *Save 15% online with the code THRIVE at https://redmond.life.*

Buying Tips

There are many fancy sea salts available, and these can be fun to experiment with when cooking. For your medicine cabinet, though, any simple sea salt without anti-caking agents is fine.

Shelf Life

Sea salt will last indefinitely, but exposure to moisture can cause it to clump.

Actions

Sea salt can act as an exfoliant and nurturing agent for the skin, as well as a disinfectant for the skin and mucous membranes.

Preparations & Dosage

Sea salt is very easy to use at home. Dosing guidelines are not needed.

- A simple saline solution is the most common way to use sea salt as a remedy.
- It can also be mixed into bath water, with or without Epsom salt and/or baking soda.
- Sea salt can be combined with enough carrier oil to make a paste, then used as a skin scrub.

Contraindications

None.

How to Make Your Own

It's very easy to make your own saline solution with sea salt.

1. Add ½ teaspoon sea salt to freshly boiled water.
2. Allow to cool, then use as an eyewash, nasal rinse, gargle, or in any other place where a saline solution is needed.
3. Use within 48 hours.

You can double the sea salt for a stronger disinfecting gargle, but the salty taste may be unpleasant.

A pinch of baking soda can be added to homemade saline solution. This is called buffered saline and is more comfortable for some people.

Tummy Tea

Digestive upsets are some of the most common home ailments. Ginger (*Zingiber officinale*), peppermint (*Mentha piperita*), chamomile (*Matricaria recutita*), spearmint (*Mentha spicata*), fennel seed (*Foeniculum vulgare*), and lemon balm (*Melissa officinalis*) are common herbs that can help. If you pay close attention, you'll see that many herbs that calm the tummy also calm the nerves.

Where to Buy

Many pharmacies and grocery stores now carry quality herbal teas. Health food stores will give you more options, as will online herbal retailers and herbalist-owned online shops. Fennel seed is widely available in the spice aisle of most grocery stores. My Wellevate list includes numerous Tummy Tea options.

Buying Tips

Herbal teas can be purchased in familiar boxes of tea bags or as loose herbal mixes. You can also purchase individual herbs separately and blend your own tea. Loose herbal tea allows you to easily see and smell the quality of herbs in the blend, though bagged herbal tea may seem more convenient. If you choose loose herbal tea, you'll need to purchase a few brewing tools like metal mesh tea strainers or reusable muslin tea bags.

Shelf Life

Dry herbal teas are best used within one year of purchase.

Actions

Specific actions will vary depending on the individual herbs in your blend, but most will have the following actions:

- *Antispasmodic*—reduces muscle spasms, cramps, and tension
- *Aromatic*—eases nausea due to volatile oil content
- *Carminative*—relieves intestinal gas and bloating

Preparations & Dosage

Chewing a few fennel seeds is one of the simplest digestive remedies. It's quite effective, too. There's no preparation needed outside of opening the container, popping a few in your mouth, and chewing away. This is safe for adults and children.

Strong herbal teas are called infusions and can be made by steeping 1-2 teaspoons dried herb (or 1-2 teabags) in 1 cup of freshly boiled water for 30 minutes in a covered mug. Strain the herbs or remove the tea bags, then sweeten with honey if desired.

Because the digestive herbs mentioned are very safe, dosing is flexible.

- Adults can take a tea up to 3-5 times daily during illness or gastrointestinal discomfort, or 1-2 cups at a time as needed.
- Children ages 7-12 can take 2 cups throughout the day, or 1 cup at a time as needed.
- Children ages 2-6 can take 1 cup of tea throughout the day, or ½ cup at a time as needed.

Contraindications

None.

How to Make Your Own

Your Relaxant Nervine tea can double as a Tummy Tea in a pinch, but I prefer keeping a blend of peppermint (*Mentha piperita*), spearmint (*Mentha spicata*), and chamomile (*Matricaria recutita*) on hand, too. Adding a slice of fresh ginger to your mug when brewing perfects the blend!

1. Measure out **1 part peppermint, 1 part spearmint, and 2 parts chamomile** in a bowl. You can measure the herbs by weight or by volume.
2. Combine the herbs completely, crushing any pieces that are substantially larger than the rest of the herb pieces.
3. Transfer to a glass jar and label with product name, herbs included, and blending date.

To use, follow the process above for brewing loose herbal infusions, adding a slice of fresh ginger to your mug before covering to steep. A squeeze of fresh lemon adds flavor and additional digestive help.

Bone, K. & Mills, S. (2013). *Principles and Practice of Phytotherapy: Modern Herbal Medicine*. London: Elsevier.

Hoffmann, D. (2003). *Medical Herbalism: The Science and Practice of Herbal Medicine*. Rochester, VT: Healing Arts Press.

Romm, A. (2018). *Botanical Medicine for Women's Health* (2nd ed.). St. Louis, MO: Elsevier.

Turmeric

Turmeric (*Curcuma longa*) is a common spice found in curry, but it's gaining well-deserved popularity for its numerous health-promoting properties. Curcumin is the important active compound that gives turmeric its rich, golden hue.

Where to Buy

Dry, powdered turmeric can be found in the spice aisle of most grocery stores. The fresh root is sometimes available in the refrigerated produce section near ginger root. Health food stores may offer more varieties of turmeric preparations, including "golden milk" mixes, turmeric capsules, and various turmeric extracts. Even more options are available from online retailers. I've included various forms of turmeric in the Wellevate list.

Buying Tips

There are many ways to take, and therefore purchase, turmeric. The simplest is to find a quality turmeric powder. It should have a rich golden color and be free from artificial dyes. It should also have a slightly pungent smell and remind you of curry.

Turmeric extracts and capsule preparations may include piperine, a compound derived from black pepper. This improves the body's ability to absorb curcumin and is a beneficial addition to these products.

Shelf Life

Powdered turmeric is best used within 6-12 months.

Actions

- *Anti-inflammatory*—reduces pain, redness, and swelling from inflammation
- *Antimutagenic/Antitumor*—promotes healthy cell replication
- *Antimicrobial*—reduces pathogenic microbes
- *Antioxidant*—reduces the effects of harmful oxidation processes
- *Digestive*—improves digestive function
- *Tonic Protective*—nourishes and protects major body systems
- *Vulnerary*—promotes wound healing

Preparations & Dosage

Turmeric may be taken to protect against illness, encourage a robust recovery from illness, and simply in cooking for taste and color. There are many preparation options:

- It can be added to stir-fries, curries, soups, stews, rice dishes, and more.
- It can be blended with warming spices, then stirred into dairy or non-dairy milk to make a health-promoting drink called "golden milk."
- It can be mixed into a paste with honey (for taste) and a small amount of oil (for bioavailability) and taken by the teaspoonful during illness.
- It can be taken in capsules if the taste is disagreeable.

An adult dose of turmeric is approximately 1 teaspoon powdered turmeric, once or twice a day. This dose can be increased during times of illness.

For children, reduce the dose as follows:

- For children ages 7-12, ½ teaspoon can be used once or twice a day.
- For children ages 2-6, ¼ teaspoon can be used once or twice a day.

Children will likely take turmeric more readily if it is paired with honey.

Contraindications

None, though high doses may be contraindicated for those with gallstones or other bile obstructions. Medicinal daily doses are not recommended during pregnancy.

How to Make Your Own

Many people enjoy drinking Golden Milk as an alternative to coffee or tea. There are various recipes available, and each can be tweaked to suit your preferences. One example is:

1. Combine 1 heaping teaspoon turmeric powder with ½ teaspoon cinnamon, ¼ teaspoon ginger powder, and ¼ teaspoon cardamom in a mug and stir to combine.
2. Heat 1 cup milk (dairy or non-dairy) in a small saucepan until hot but not boiling, and pour into the mug.
3. Stir until no clumps of spice remain, then add honey to taste.

This can be taken daily, or whenever you want an anti-inflammatory drink.

There may be some sediment at the bottom of your mug with this method. To avoid too much sediment, stir your Golden Milk occasionally while drinking. If this bothers you, you can mix the spices with the hot milk in a measuring cup, then pour into a mug through a fine-mesh sieve before drinking.

Bone, K. & Mills, S. (2013). *Principles and Practice of Phytotherapy: Modern Herbal Medicine*. London: Elsevier.

Engles, G. (2009). Turmeric. *HerbalGram* (84), 1-3. Retrieved from http://cms.herbalgram.org/herbalgram/issue84/article3450.html.

Romm, A. (2017). The Adrenal Thyroid Revolution: A Proven 4-Week Program to Rescue Your Metabolism, Hormones, Mind, & Mood. New York, NY: HarperOne.

Turmeric. (n.d.). *Healthy Ingredients*. Retrieved from http://cms.herbalgram.org/healthyingredients/Turmeric.html.

Turmeric Root. (2000). *Herbal Medicine: Expanded Commission E*. Retrieved from http://cms.herbalgram.org/expandedE/Turmericroot.html.

Turmeric Root. (1990). *The Commission E Monographs*. Retrieved from http://cms.herbalgram.org/commissione/Monographs/Monograph0361.html.

Witch Hazel

Witch hazel (*Hamamelis virginiana*) is a shrub native to the USA. Its bark, leaf, and twigs are used medicinally. The most common preparation, and what you can stock in your natural medicine cabinet, is the clear distilled extract made from witch hazel twigs.

Where to Buy

Witch hazel distillate, the familiar clear liquid, is available in most grocery stores and pharmacies near the rubbing alcohol, hydrogen peroxide, and other first-aid supplies.

Buying Tips

Most witch hazels include 14% alcohol as a preservative. There are some alcohol-free options available, but these will contain other preservatives like citric acid and grapefruit seed extract. Standard witch hazel distillates with alcohol are perfectly fine for your medicine cabinet, but if your skin is sensitive to the alcohol content you can try an alcohol-free version.

Shelf Life

Witch hazel distillate will last for years, but check the expiration date on your bottle for a precise shelf life.

Actions

- *Analgesic*—reduces pain
- *Anti-inflammatory*—reduces pain, redness, and swelling from inflammation
- *Astringent*—tones and tightens tissue
- *Vulnerary*—promotes wound healing

Preparations & Dosage

Witch hazel is an excellent remedy for topical concerns such as rashes, cuts, acne, bruises, varicose veins, and more. It does not need to be rinsed off and can be applied multiple times a day if needed.

- It can be applied to the face after washing as a toner.
- It can be applied to pimples to reduce redness and swelling.
- It can be widely applied to skin irritations from insect bites, poison ivy, and other irritants throughout the day as needed.
- It can be used to speed the healing of cuts, abrasions, and bruises.
- It can be applied to tighten varicose veins.

Contraindications

None, but excessive use may result in itchy or dry skin due to the alcohol content of most witch hazel distillates. On sensitive skin or with children, witch hazel may be diluted in equal parts water.

Bone, K. & Mills, S. (2013). *Principles and Practice of Phytotherapy: Modern Herbal Medicine.* London: Elsevier.

Hoffmann, D. (2003). *Medical Herbalism: The Science and Practice of Herbal Medicine.* Rochester, VT: Healing Arts Press.

Witch Hazel Leaf and Bark. (2000). *Herbal Medicine: The Expanded Commission E.* Retrieved from http://cms.herbalgram.org/expandedE/WitchHazelleafandbark.html.

Witch Hazel Leaf and Bark. (1990). *The Commission E Monographs.* Retrieved from http://cms.herbalgram.org/commissione/Monographs/Monograph0377.html.

Part 3:
Common Ailments

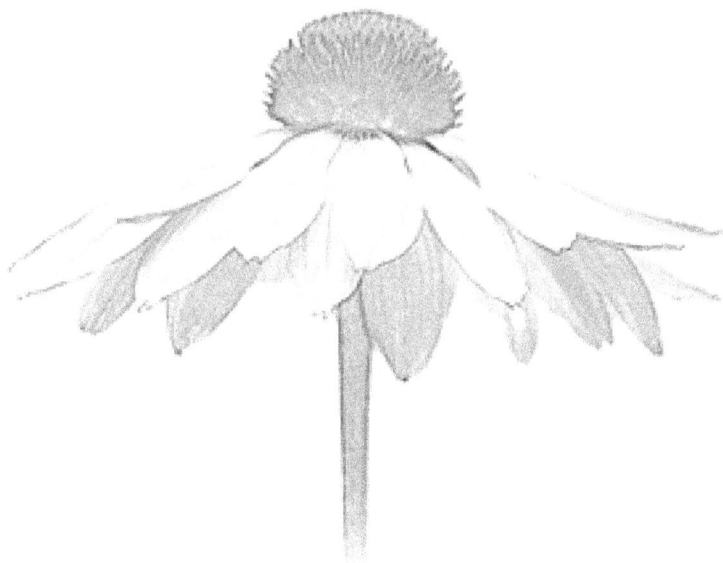

Many common ailments can be safely treated at home. The remedies in your Minimalist Natural Medicine Cabinet can support your body's natural healing mechanisms, relieve symptoms, and often get you back to your old self without a trip to the doctor.

This section covers some of the most common ailments you're likely to experience from time to time and what you can use to support health. These are listed in alphabetical order, like the Remedies are, with the following information provided:

- *Potential Root Causes* offers a starting place for understanding why an ailment occurred.
- *Minimalist Natural Medicine Cabinet Remedies* lists remedies from the previous section which can help that ailment.
- *Specific Remedies* gives you additional remedy options that may be worth stocking. If you or someone in your house is prone to a certain ailment, it may be wise to stock some specific remedies that offer additional support.

Sometimes it can be difficult to know which remedies to use if multiple concerns are going on at once or other complicating factors. During those times, it helps to talk with a natural health professional who works one-on-one with clients.

As an herbalist and aromatherapist, I would be happy to help you work towards your health and wellness goals. You can learn about my client work at https://abetterwaytothrive.com/services/thriving-health-consultations.

Also, remember there's no shame in visiting your licensed healthcare provider when needed. Even if you prefer using natural remedies instead of pharmaceutical products, a doctor or nurse practitioner can provide you with valuable information, guidance, and yes, sometimes treatments, that will help you recover completely.

Unless otherwise noted, references for this section include:

Bone, K. & Mills, S. (2013). *Principles and Practice of Phytotherapy: Modern Herbal Medicine.* London: Elsevier.

Hoffmann, D. (2003). *Medical Herbalism: The Science and Practice of Herbal Medicine.* Rochester, VT: Healing Arts Press.

Price, S. & Price, P. (2012). *Aromatherapy for Health Professionals* (4th ed.). London: Elsevier.

Romm, A. (2018). *Botanical Medicine for Women's Health* (2nd ed.). St. Louis, MO: Elsevier.

Acne/Blemishes

Acne and blemishes can be embarrassing and cause emotional and mental distress. Natural remedies can be as effective as some pharmaceutical products, especially when root causes are considered and addressed.

Potential Root Causes

- Hormonal imbalances and/or shifts
- Gut flora imbalances (dysbiosis)
- Inflammatory foods or food sensitivities

Minimalist Natural Medicine Cabinet Remedies

- Witch hazel can be applied with a cotton ball as a toner in between washing and moisturizing. It can also be used as a spot treatment.
- Lavender and tea tree essential oil can be added to a light carrier oil at a 2% dilution and used as a moisturizer after washing. A 5% dilution can be used as a spot treatment.
- Bentonite clay can be hydrated with equal parts honey and water until a paste forms, then applied over the affected area as a mask. This can be rinsed off after 15 minutes.
- Bentonite clay paste can also be used as an overnight spot treatment and rinsed off in the morning.
- Honey can be applied to blemishes at night before going to bed as a spot treatment.
- Healing salve can be applied over areas that feel dry.

Specific Remedies

- Liver supportive herbs can help the body process excess hormones. Milk thistle (*Silybum marianum*) and dandelion root (*Taraxacum officinale*) are two common liver herbs.
- Probiotic supplements and/or fermented foods can encourage healthy gut flora.

Allergies (Seasonal)

Allergy treatment varies from person to person, depending on the type of allergy. These remedies provide a starting place.

Potential Root Causes

- Gut flora imbalances (dysbiosis)
- Poor air quality due to pollen

Minimalist Natural Medicine Cabinet Remedies

- Raw, local honey can be taken daily before and during allergy season to reduce symptoms and normalize the immune response.
- Sea salt can be made into a saline solution and used 1-2 times daily as a nasal rinse to clear out excess pollen from nasal passages and reduce sinus congestion.
- Lavender essential oil can be inhaled throughout the day to reduce inflammation of the eyes, nose, and throat.
- Eucalyptus essential oil can be inhaled or diluted and applied topically to promote clear breathing. Peppermint may also be used with adults.
- Cold and Flu Relief tea may provide symptomatic relief.

Specific Remedies

Three additional herbs are often used in allergy formulas:

- Nettles (*Urtica dioica*)
- Eyebright (*Euphrasia officinalis*)
- Goldenrod (*Solidago virgaurea*)

These herbs can be taken daily as very strong infusions or as tinctures.

Along with these herbs, fermented foods and/or probiotic supplements can improve gut flora and regulate the immune response.

Bruises, Sprains, & Strains

Sports activities, exercise, yard work, and physically demanding jobs can all contribute to bruises and other soft tissue injuries. Mild injuries can be treated at home with the following remedies, but always seek medical care for injuries that significantly interfere with daily life activities.

Potential Root Causes

- Trauma
- Overwork
- Injury

Minimalist Natural Medicine Cabinet Remedies

- Epsom salt baths, with or without properly diluted lavender essential oil, can soothe and nourish tired muscles.
- Arnica, either homeopathic or topical, can reduce pain, swelling, and bruising when used multiple times a day until symptoms are reduced.
- Healing salve can be applied over the area for localized relief.
- Peppermint and/or lavender essential oil can be properly diluted and topically applied for pain relief.
- Turmeric can be taken to ease inflammation from injury.

Specific Remedies

Rest, ice, compression, and elevation (when applicable) are tried and true remedies that can also be included.

Bug Bites & Stings

Bug bites and stings can be painful and often result in itchy welts. Quick treatment can speed healing and reduce discomfort.

Potential Root Causes

- Insect exposure

Minimalist Natural Medicine Cabinet Remedies

- Baking soda can be mixed with water to form a paste and applied to painful stings and bites. This can be reapplied as needed.
- Lavender essential oil can be diluted and topically applied over the affected area to ease inflammation and itching.
- Healing salve can be applied to bites and stings as they heal.
- Witch hazel can be applied over affected areas as needed to reduce inflammation.

Specific Remedies

Plantain (*Plantago major*) is a common yard weed that can be quickly used as a sting or bite remedy when outside. A single leaf can be chewed, then applied to the sting or bite until the pain stops. Though this spit poultice is a very "rustic" remedy, it's also very effective!

Burns

Burns can be painful and lead to blistering. Promptly caring for burns with simple natural remedies can protect against further problems. *Always seek medical care for severe burns.*

Potential Root Causes

- Excessive sun exposure
- Excessive heat exposure
- Other irritant exposure

Minimalist Natural Medicine Cabinet Remedies

- Aloe gel, either bottled or fresh, can be applied to the burn multiple times a day as needed to reduce inflammation and encourage healing.
- Healing salve can be applied as needed after blisters go down to promote skin regeneration.
- Lavender essential oil can be diluted and applied to reduce inflammation and speed healing. A drop of lavender can be immediately applied neat (undiluted) on adults to the affected area after mild kitchen burns.
- Honey can be applied topically, then covered with a bandage, to encourage healing and protect against infection.
- Turmeric can be taken internally to reduce inflammation.

Specific Remedies

Hydrosols are distilled herbal waters and offer many benefits to the skin. The following hydrosols can be especially soothing to burns:

- Rose (*Rosa damascena*)
- Calendula (*Calendula officinalis*)
- Chamomile (*Matricaria recutita*)
- Cucumber (*Cucumis sativus*)
- Peppermint (*Mentha piperita*)

Constipation

Constipation can be an uncomfortable issue, especially for children. While diet and lifestyle adjustments often take care of constipation, additional remedies can provide extra support.

Potential Root Causes

- Gut flora imbalances (dysbiosis)
- Dehydration
- Lack of dietary fiber
- Lack of physical movement and exercise
- Stress
- Magnesium deficiency

Minimalist Natural Medicine Cabinet Remedies

- Relaxing Nervine Tea can be taken as needed if constipation is tied to stress. This will also encourage better hydration.
- Tummy Tea can be taken as needed to improve hydration and promote digestion.
- Apple cider vinegar can be taken in water 15-30 minutes before eating to promote digestion.
- Sweet orange essential oil can be inhaled before and after eating to promote digestion and relaxation.
- Epsom salts can be used in a bath to promote relaxation and gently increase magnesium levels.

Specific Remedies

Dietary changes and nutritional supplements should be the first place to start when dealing with constipation.

- Dietary fiber can be increased by eating more fruits and vegetables at every meal.
- Probiotic supplements and/or fermented foods can be taken to improve gut flora.

- Magnesium supplementation with magnesium citrate or glycinate can promote regular bowel movements.
- Increased water intake and decreased consumption of caffeinated beverages (coffee, soda, black/green tea, etc.) can improve hydration, which in turn reduces constipation.

Herbal bitters can be taken by adults before meals to stimulate digestion and intestinal peristalsis (the muscle movements needed to produce a bowel movement). These are taken as extracts and often include the following herbs:

- Burdock (*Arctium lappa*)
- Dandelion root (*Taraxacum officinale*)
- Chicory (*Cichorium intybus*)
- Orange peel (*Citrus sinensis* or *C. aurantium*)
- Fennel (*Foeniculum vulgare*)

Some herbs reduce constipation by acting as mild, bulk laxatives or gentle stimulant laxatives. Some final herbs to consider are:

- Psyllium (*Plantago psyllium*) and flax (*Linum usitatissimum*) seeds are bulk laxatives. These can be taken ground, with plenty of water, 1-3 times a day until constipation resolves.
- Senna (*Senna alexandrina*) is a stimulant laxative that can be used occasionally by non-pregnant adults.
- Marshmallow root (*Althaea officinalis*) and slippery elm bark (*Ulmus rubra*) contain slippery mucilage which can soothe the digestive tract and reduce constipation. These are best taken as powders with plenty of water.

Coughs

Coughs can be wet or dry, nagging or occasional, chronic or acute, and due to several root causes. When considering remedies for a cough, think through the specifics of the cough and how to best support healing.

Potential Root Causes

- Bacterial or viral infections
- Allergies
- Exposure to irritants
- Gastrointestinal reflux
- Pharmaceutical medications

Minimalist Natural Medicine Cabinet Remedies

- One teaspoon honey can be taken as a simple cough syrup as needed.
- Sliced garlic cloves can be covered in honey for 12-24 hours, then strained out. The garlic honey can be taken by the teaspoon as a cough syrup.
- Lemon and honey can be added to a strong ginger infusion and taken as needed throughout the day to relieve nagging coughs.
- Cold and Flu Relief Tea can be taken if the underlying cause is an infection, with honey added for additional cough relief.
- Eucalyptus essential oil can be inhaled and/or diluted and topically applied to the chest to assist wet coughs.
- Relaxing Nervine Tea can be taken 1-3 times a day for nagging, dry coughs.
- Sea salt can be made into a saline solution and used as a gargle and nasal rinse.

Specific Remedies

- Mullein leaf (*Verbascum thapsus*) strengthens and soothes the respiratory system. It can be made into an infusion and taken with honey 1-3 times a day.
- Marshmallow root (*Althaea officinalis*) or slippery elm bark (*Ulmus rubra*) powder can be mixed with honey to form a thick paste. This paste can then be rolled into small lozenges, left to dry overnight, and used as simple cough drops to soothe irritated tissue.
- Hyssop (*Hyssopus officinalis*) is antispasmodic and expectorant, so it can be used with wet, nagging coughs. It can be taken as an infusion or tincture.
- Wild cherry bark (*Prunus serotina*) calms the cough reflex and can be especially useful at night when coughing prevents sleep. It can be taken as a tincture and is sometimes included in herbal cough drops.

Cuts & Scratches

Cuts and scratches are part of everyday life, especially for children. These can be easily remedied with your Minimalist Natural Medicine Cabinet.

Potential Root Causes

- Accidents

Minimalist Natural Medicine Cabinet Remedies

- Witch hazel can be applied over the affected area after initial cleaning and before applying a salve and bandage.
- Healing salve can be applied over the cut before bandaging to encourage quick healing, reduce the risk of infection, and reduce pain and inflammation. *Seek medical treatment before applying a healing salve over a deep cut which may need stitches.*
- Lavender and/or tea tree oil can be diluted and applied topically to encourage healing and reduce the risk of infection.

Specific Remedies

Hydrosols, mentioned earlier under Burns, can also be used for cuts and scratches to encourage healing. The following hydrosols are well-suited:

- Calendula (*Calendula officinalis*)
- Lavender (*Lavandula angustifolia*)
- Rose (*Rosa damascena*)
- Chamomile (*Matricaria recutita*)

Diarrhea

Most often, diarrhea needs to simply run its course over a couple of days to resolve. But it can be uncomfortable and lead to dehydration in children, justifying the use of some natural remedies.

Potential Root Causes

- Stress
- Infection
- Exposure to foodborne pathogens
- Food intolerance or sensitivity
- Gut flora imbalances (dysbiosis)

Minimalist Natural Medicine Cabinet Remedies

- Tummy Tea can be brewed into a strong infusion with a slice of ginger and taken 3-5 times a day while symptoms last.
- A simple rehydration drink can be made with lemon, honey, and a pinch of sea salt in a glass of water to ward off dehydration from diarrhea.
- If the diarrhea is due to infection, elderberry syrup or gummies can be taken 3-5 times a day, along with echinacea extract.
- Sweet orange essential oil can be inhaled throughout the day to promote healthy digestive function.

Specific Remedies

- Bananas, applesauce, white rice, cooked potatoes, and yogurt (if dairy isn't a food sensitivity) are easily digested foods that can slow diarrhea.
- Probiotic supplements or fermented foods and drinks can promote healthy gut microbial balance during and after diarrhea.
- A strong infusion of blackberry leaf or root (*Rubus fruticosus*) can tone and tighten intestinal tissue, reducing symptoms of diarrhea.

Dry Skin

Dry skin can happen seasonally, from aging, or as a result of other exposures. Most remedies will focus on topical treatment, but some internal remedies and supplements can assist in healing, also.

Potential Root Causes

- Aging
- Dry indoor air during cold seasons
- Repeat hand washing
- Exposure to irritants

Minimalist Natural Medicine Cabinet Remedies

- A carrier oil can be applied to damp hands after washing to seal in moisture.
- Lavender essential oil can be diluted in a carrier and applied at night before bed.
- Sea salt, honey, and a carrier oil can be blended into a thin paste and used as a scrub, then rinsed off. Lavender or orange essential oil can also be added.
- Healing salve can be applied to painful, dry skin, especially if the skin is flaking or cracking.
- Aloe gel can be applied and allowed to dry on the skin, followed by a carrier oil or healing salve.

Specific Remedies

- Hard lotion bars are especially helpful for dry skin of the hands, feet, elbows, and knees. These are made of oil (like coconut), butter (like shea), and beeswax, and can be applied to the skin in place of liquid lotion.
- Omega-3 fatty acid supplements, like cod liver oil, can promote healthy skin.
- Unscented soaps can prevent irritation.
- A nutrient-rich diet with ample hydration can improve overall skin health.

Earaches

Earache treatment generally focuses on symptom relief while the condition resolves on its own. Earaches and ear infections don't require antibiotics every time, but a ruptured eardrum is grounds for a trip to your licensed healthcare provider.

Potential Root Causes

- Fluid congestion in the inner ear from a respiratory infection
- Dairy intolerance

Minimalist Natural Medicine Cabinet Remedies

- A garlic clove can be minced and warmed in 1 tablespoon carrier oil for 30 minutes, then strained. A few drops of the warm garlic-infused oil can be poured in the ear for pain relief and antimicrobial benefits. A cotton ball can be placed over the ear to catch any excess oil. *Do not use ear oil if the eardrum has ruptured.*
- Echinacea extract can be given at appropriate doses to help fight infection.
- Cold & Flu Relief Tea can be taken throughout the day to boost immune response and help with congestion.
- Turmeric can be mixed with honey to form a thin paste and taken by the teaspoon to reduce pain and inflammation.
- Lavender essential oil can be diluted and applied around the ear for pain relief. *Do not put essential oils in the ear.*
- Eucalyptus essential oil can be diluted and applied topically to the chest to encourage clearer breathing and help loosen congested mucus.
- Sea salt can be made into a saline solution and used as a nasal rinse to clear underlying congestion.

Specific Remedies

- Mullein flower (*Verbascum thapsus*) can be added to the garlic when making a garlic ear oil. There are also many quality ear oil products on the market which contain both of these herbs.
- Chiropractic care can provide relief by promoting proper drainage of the inner ear tubes.
- Some children who have recurring ear infections and earaches may have an underlying dairy sensitivity. Dairy can be removed from the diet for 2-4 weeks, then reintroduced to observe the response, if dairy is a suspected trigger.
- Probiotics and/or fermented foods and drinks can be given to children who have taken antibiotics for earaches and ear infections to restore healthy gut flora.

Fatigue

Fatigue is generally the body's way of telling us it needs attention. Finding the root cause of fatigue is necessary to know how to treat it.

Potential Root Causes

- Overwork
- Stress
- Sleep disturbances
- Sleep deprivation
- Recovery from infection, injury, or surgery
- Dehydration
- Growth spurts (children)
- Pregnancy
- Hypothyroidism

Minimalist Natural Medicine Cabinet Remedies

- Daily Epsom salt baths can be taken in the evenings, with or without lavender essential oil diluted in 1 teaspoon *each* carrier oil and liquid soap, to promote restful sleep and better energy.
- Relaxing Nervine Tea can be taken every night to promote better sleep and reduce stress levels.
- Lavender and sweet orange essential oils can be inhaled nightly before bed to promote restful sleep. A drop of one or both can also be put on a tissue, then tucked under the pillowcase before going to bed.
- A drop of peppermint essential oil can be placed on a cotton ball or tissue and inhaled for 10-15 minutes to energize the mind and body during the day. A drop of sweet orange or lavender can be added according to preference.
- Lemon water can be drunk when fatigued as an alternative to caffeinated or sugary drinks.
- Tummy Tea, with its invigorating mints, can be taken when fatigued instead of caffeinated or sugary drinks.

Specific Remedies

- Earlier bedtimes and/or afternoon naps can provide more energy and give the body required extra rest.
- Appropriate exercise can naturally boost energy. Daily walks outside are an excellent choice for many people.
- Peppermint and nettle infusion is a nourishing, invigorating drink that can be enjoyed in the afternoon when fatigue often sets in. It is delicious hot or chilled and with or without lemon.
- Rosemary (*Rosmarinus officinalis* ct Cineole or Camphor) essential oil can be inhaled on its own or with peppermint and/or sweet orange to stimulate mental energy and clear thinking. *Rosemary is contraindicated in seizure disorders*.

Fever

It is almost always better to work with fevers than it is to fight them. These remedies can help with the pain often associated with fever and regulate fever levels. *Fevers in newborns and very high fevers require medical attention.*

Potential Root Causes

- Infection
- Excessive heat exposure

Minimalist Natural Medicine Cabinet Remedies

- Cold & Flu Relief Tea can be taken throughout the day as needed to regulate the fever.
- Lavender essential oil can be diluted and applied topically along the forehead and back of the neck to relieve fever discomfort in young children.
- Peppermint essential oil can be diluted and applied topically along the forehead and back of the neck to relieve fever discomfort in older children and adults.
- Ginger can be brewed into a strong tea or decoction and taken throughout the day to help regulate fever.
- Garlic can be taken to encourage sweating and healthy fever levels, and also fight off infection.
- Honey can be added to herbal teas to provide the body needed energy and help fight off infection.
- Epsom salt baths can be taken, with or without properly diluted lavender essential oil, to relieve fever discomfort and regulate fever. Bathwater should be comfortably warm, but not hot or cold.
- Turmeric can be mixed with honey and a little oil to form a thin paste, then taken throughout the day to reduce painful inflammation.
- Echinacea extract and/or elderberry syrup or gummies can be taken to help fight off infection.

Specific Remedies

- Willow (*Salix alba*), an anti-inflammatory and analgesic herb, can be used to gently lower fevers when needed and to reduce pain. It is often taken as a tincture.

Fungal Skin Infections (Tinea Infections)

Tinea infections are fungal skin infections that commonly occur on the feet (Athlete's foot, or Tinea pedis), groin (jock itch, or Tinea cruris), and other parts of the body (ringworm, or Tinea corporis). Depending on the location, fungal skin infections can resolve quickly or be quite stubborn.

Potential Root Causes

- Poor airflow and excess moisture on affected skin (sweaty socks, shoes, underwear, etc. kept on for too long)
- Gut flora imbalances (dysbiosis)
- Weak immune system
- Recent antibiotic use

Minimalist Natural Medicine Cabinet Remedies

- Witch hazel can be applied topically to weeping fungal infections as needed.
- Garlic can be added liberally to the diet to improve immune function and gut flora. Garlic can also be infused in apple cider vinegar, carrier oil, or honey and used as suggested below. Crush the peeled cloves, cover with vinegar, oil, or honey, then set in a warm place to infuse for at least 3 hours, or overnight. Strain and refrigerate the final product.
- Apple cider vinegar can be diluted in water (1-2 tablespoons vinegar per cup of water) and used as a topical wash or soak over affected areas 1-3 times per day.
- Tea tree oil can be diluted in a carrier oil (2-5 drops per teaspoon of carrier oil) and applied over affected areas 1-3 times per day and after apple cider vinegar soaks. Lavender essential oil can be used along with or in place of tea tree oil.
- Honey can be applied over affected areas overnight, covered with a cloth or light bandage.
- Healing salve can be applied over dry, cracked, or peeling skin.
- Echinacea extract can be taken to improve the immune response.

Specific Remedies

- Eliminating or greatly reducing sugar consumption (including refined flour) can improve immune function and gut flora balance.
- Exposing the affected areas to airflow and sunlight, if possible, can speed healing.
- Oregon grape root (*Mahonia aquifolium*) is an antifungal herb. The tincture can be taken internally for stubborn Tinea infections.

Stansbury, Jill. (2018). *Herbal Formularies for Health Professionals: Digestion and Elimination.* Chelsea Green Publishing: White River Junction, VT.

Gas & Bloating

Gas and abdominal bloating after meals can be very embarrassing and uncomfortable. While it's important to uncover the specific root cause to reduce situations of gas and bloating, some natural remedies can offer helpful, quick relief when they do occur.

Potential Root Causes
- Stress and anxiety
- Food intolerances and allergies
- Sleep deprivation
- Gut flora imbalances (dysbiosis)
- Infection

Minimalist Natural Medicine Cabinet Remedies
- Tummy Tea can be taken after meals or as soon as gas and bloating become apparent.
- Ginger can be taken as a strong infusion or decoction after meals or when symptoms arise.
- Peppermint or orange essential oil can be inhaled from a cotton ball, tissue, or directly from the bottle for 10-15 minutes to encourage healthy digestion.
- Strong lemon water can be taken before a meal to encourage healthy digestion and help protect against gas and bloating.
- One tablespoon apple cider vinegar can be taken in a small cup of water before a meal to encourage healthy digestion and protect against gas and bloating.

Specific Remedies

- Herbal bitters can be taken before or after a meal to encourage healthy digestion and reduce gas and bloating. These are blends of bitter, digestion-stimulating herbs that are taken as tinctures.
- An elimination diet can help uncover food intolerances that may be causing gas and bloating.
- Probiotic supplements and/or fermented foods and drinks can promote healthy gut flora and help reduce gas and bloating.

Growing Pains

Growing pains can be very uncomfortable for some children and difficult for their parents when the children wake up at night from the discomfort. While the cause and physiology aren't fully understood, some remedies can offer relief.

Potential Root Causes

- Growth spurts
- Possible nutrient deficiencies

Minimalist Natural Medicine Cabinet Remedies

- Lavender and peppermint essential oils can be diluted together in a carrier (1-2 drops *each* in 1 teaspoon carrier oil) and massaged over the painful area.
- Arnica can be taken homeopathically or used topically.
- Epsom salt baths can be taken regularly to encourage healthy muscle tone and promote relaxation.
- Relaxing Nervine Tea can be taken nightly to reduce muscle spasms and encourage restfulness.

Specific Remedies

- Vitamin D and/or magnesium supplementation may offer some benefit.
- Passionflower (*Passiflora incarnata*) can be taken in extract form while symptoms present to encourage relaxation and quick return to sleep.
- Gentle stretches can be done nightly before bed to lengthen muscles that may be excessively tight.

Lehman, P. J. & Carl, R. L. (2017). Growing pains: When to be concerned. *Sports Health, 9(2)*. 132-138. doi:10.1177/1941738117692533.

Vehapoglu, A., Turel, O., Turkmen, S., Inal, B.B., Aksoy, T., Ozgurhan, G., & Ersoy, M. (2015). Are growing pains related to Vitamin D deficiency? Efficacy of Vitamin D therapy for resolution of symptoms. *Medical Principles and Practice, 24(4)*. 332-338. doi:10.1159/000431035.

Headaches

Most people experience headaches from time to time. They can be simply annoying and mildly bothersome to debilitating and excruciating. Natural remedies offer various levels of support. As always, uncovering the root causes will be extremely valuable.

Potential Root Causes

- Magnesium deficiency
- Stress and tension
- Infection
- Sleep deprivation
- Injury
- Hormonal shifts, either cyclic or age-related
- Weather shifts
- Dehydration
- Hunger
- Artificial food additives

Minimalist Natural Medicine Cabinet Remedies

- Peppermint essential oil, with or without additional lavender and/or eucalyptus essential oil, can be diluted and applied topically to painful areas. A 3% dilution is suitable for children, pregnant women, and the elderly. Adults may find relief from 5-10% dilutions.
- If the headache seems linked to dehydration, a simple rehydration drink can be made from lemon juice, honey, and a pinch of sea salt.
- An Epsom salt bath can help reduce muscle tension and relieve stress. Lavender essential oil can be diluted in 1 teaspoon carrier oil and 1 teaspoon liquid soap, then added for additional benefit.
- Relaxing Nervine Tea can be taken to help calm muscle tension and reduce stress.
- Echinacea extract, elderberry syrup/gummies, and turmeric can be taken if the headache is due to infection or fever.

Specific Remedies

- Magnesium supplementation is often beneficial for chronic migraines or headaches. Magnesium glycinate is a well-tolerated and easily absorbed form.
- If headaches are hormone-related, chaste tree (*Vitex agnus castus*) can help regulate healthy female hormone levels. Chaste tree is also known as vitex.
- Cayenne (*Capsicum annuum*) can reduce sensitivity in pain receptors. It can be taken in capsules or with food during a headache. Topical preparations are also available and should be used with care to avoid the eyes, sensitive skin, and mucous membranes.

Heartburn & Indigestion

Heartburn occurs when stomach contents come back up through the esophagus after eating. Indigestion is sometimes synonymous with heartburn; other times it simply refers to sluggish digestion.

Potential Root Causes

- Pregnancy
- Stress
- Food intolerances or sensitivities
- Pharmaceutical medications
- Smoking
- Alcohol use
- Processed foods

Minimalist Natural Medicine Cabinet Remedies

- Apple cider vinegar mixed with water can be taken 15-30 minutes before eating to promote healthy digestion.
- Tummy tea can be taken when symptoms present to encourage digestion and soothe digestive muscle spasms.
- Peppermint essential oil and/or sweet orange essential oil can be inhaled for 10-15 minutes to encourage digestion.
- Ginger can be brewed into a strong infusion or decoction and taken when symptoms present.
- Lemon can be squeezed into water and taken 15-30 minutes before a meal. It can be taken in a small amount of water after a meal when symptoms present.

Specific Remedies

- Herbal bitters can be taken by adults before meals to promote healthy digestion.
- Digestive enzyme supplements can provide additional digestive support if the above remedies don't provide relief.
- A healthy lifestyle with nutrient-rich foods, no smoking, and little to no alcohol use can protect against heartburn and indigestion.
- If a medication seems linked to heartburn or indigestion, speak with the prescribing care provider.

Immune System Support

Certain times of the year tend to leave us more prone to illness, such as the post-holiday season in January. Some remedies can boost immune system function and help protect against illnesses when you feel you may be at greater risk.

Potential Root Causes

- Sleep deprivation
- Excess sugar in the diet
- Stress
- Lack of time spent outdoors

Minimalist Natural Medicine Cabinet Remedies

- Elderberry preparations are the classic immune-boosting remedy. Elderberry can be taken daily as a preventative remedy or multiple times a day during sickness.
- Tea tree essential oil can be inhaled 10-15 minutes per day, as well as added to homemade cleaning products.
- Garlic and ginger can be added liberally to the diet.
- Honey can be taken to encourage a healthy immune response.

Specific Remedies

- Fire cider is a folk remedy created by herbalist Rosemary Gladstar. Recipes vary, but the loose formulation includes garlic, ginger, onion, horseradish, hot peppers, and any other pungent herbs infused in raw apple cider vinegar. Honey is added to taste after straining the herbs. It can be taken similarly to elderberry syrup: daily for immune support, multiple times a day during infection.
- Vitamin C and Vitamin D supplementation may help support the immune system and protect against illness.
- Astragalus (*Astragalus membranaceus*) is an adaptogenic herb often used as an immune system tonic. It can be taken daily for immune support in tinctures or strong decoctions.

Insomnia & Restlessness

Difficulty sleeping can be frustrating and lead to feeling chronically tired. It can also wear down immunity, potentially leading to more sickness. Remedies that promote good rest can also improve overall health and wellness.

Potential Root Causes

- Strong emotions, like anxiety, grief, nervousness, or anger
- Nutrient deficiencies, such as low iron or magnesium
- Caffeine-containing foods and drinks
- Hormonal shifts or imbalances

Minimalist Natural Medicine Cabinet Remedies

- Relaxing Nervine Tea can be taken nightly before bed to promote good rest.
- Epsom salt baths can be taken regularly to reduce stress.
- Lavender and sweet orange essential oils can be used topically (diluted), through inhalation, and in bath water (diluted in a carrier oil and liquid soap) to promote restfulness. A drop can be added to a tissue and tucked under the pillowcase to provide an aromatherapy treatment through the night.

Specific Remedies

- Magnesium supplementation can promote relaxation and reduce muscle tension and spasms that make it difficult to sleep.
- Iron supplementation can improve sleep quality if anemia is a problem.
- Regular exercise at least 3 hours before bedtime can improve sleep quality at night.
- Reducing screen exposure at night can encourage better quality sleep and reduce the time it takes to fall asleep.
- Journaling can help process difficult emotions so that sleep can be improved.
- Eliminating caffeine after 3 pm can reduce restlessness and improve sleep quality.

Joint Pain

Joint pain may be due to arthritic conditions, injury, age, infection, or other causes. Natural remedies include both topical and internal preparations that can help address root causes and provide local, symptomatic relief.

Potential Root Causes

- Inflammation due to injury or infection
- Age-related arthritis
- Inflammatory arthritis
- Food intolerances or sensitivities
- Artificial food additives

Minimalist Natural Medicine Cabinet Remedies

- Epsom salt baths can be taken regularly to nourish irritated tissue.
- Peppermint essential oil can be diluted and applied topically to provide pain relief. Lavender and/or eucalyptus essential oils can also be included.
- Arnica can be used to reduce pain and inflammation, either topically or homeopathically.
- Turmeric can be taken daily to reduce pain and inflammation.
- Ginger can be brewed into a strong infusion or decoction and taken daily. Lemon and honey can be added for taste and nutrients.
- Ginger can be shredded and made into a strong infusion. The shredded root can be placed in a cloth, then soaked in the infusion, and applied topically to promote circulation and improve mobility.

Specific Remedies

Specific remedies for joint pain will vary depending on the type of pain and the root cause.

- A diet rich in fruits and vegetables can decrease inflammation and overall pain levels.
- Switching from regular or diet sodas to water with lemon can reduce joint pain for some individuals, particularly those with inflammatory arthritic conditions.
- Willow (*Salix alba*) can be taken as a tincture or other extract to reduce pain.
- Dandelion leaf (*Taraxacum officinale*) can be added liberally to the diet or taken as a strong infusion to promote healthy detoxification and elimination of excess fluids.

Menstrual Cramps

Menstrual cramps are more than just a regular nuisance for many women; they can interrupt life and make regular activities impossible. Natural remedies can help with the symptoms while some lifestyle changes can reduce overall severity.

Potential Root Causes

- Hormonal shifts
- Nutrient deficiencies

Minimalist Natural Medicine Cabinet Remedies

- Lavender essential oil can be diluted and applied topically to the abdomen to reduce pain and promote relaxation.
- Ginger can be brewed into a strong infusion or decoction and taken daily to improve pelvic circulation.
- Epsom salt baths can be taken daily to reduce muscle cramps. Lavender essential oil can be diluted in a carrier oil and liquid soap, then added to the bath for additional benefits.
- Relaxing Nervine Tea can be taken daily to reduce muscle cramps, spasms, and tension and improve rest.

Specific Remedies

- Chaste berry (*Vitex agnus castus*) can help balance hormones and reduce menstrual cramping. It can be taken as a tincture.
- Cramp bark (*Viburnum opulus*) and black haw (*Viburnum prunifolium*) are often found in herbal formulas for menstrual discomfort and pain. They can be taken alone, together, or with other herbs and are most easily taken as a tincture.
- Magnesium glycinate supplementation can reduce menstrual pain and other symptoms.
- Yarrow (*Achillea millefolium*) can be taken as an infusion or a tincture and can be particularly helpful if menstrual cramps are accompanied with heavy bleeding.

- A diet rich in fruits and vegetables can lower overall inflammation and ease menstrual discomforts.
- Milk thistle seed (*Silybum marianum*) and dandelion root (*Taraxacum officinale*) support the liver and can help the body better process shifting hormones.
- Clary sage (*Salvia sclarea*) essential oil can be inhaled 1-2 times a day during menstruation and/or diluted and applied topically to the abdomen.

Muscle Pain

Muscle pain is usually due to exercise soreness, overwork, or injury, making topical remedies the most helpful choice.

Potential Root Causes

- Exercise or activity soreness
- Overwork
- Injury

Minimalist Natural Medicine Cabinet Remedies

- Epsom salt baths, either localized soaks or full body baths, can be taken daily until the soreness subsides.
- Lavender, eucalyptus, and/or peppermint essential oils can be diluted in a carrier oil and massaged over the sore muscles. These can be used alone or in any pleasing combination, diluted to about 5 total drops in 1 teaspoon carrier oil for adults.
- Arnica can be taken homeopathically or topically to reduce pain.
- Turmeric can be taken to reduce inflammation if the muscles are especially sore and painful after an injury.
- Relaxing Nervine Tea can be taken throughout the day if painful muscles feel cramped or spastic.

Specific Remedies

- Chiropractic care and professional massage treatments can provide deeper relief for chronic muscle pain.
- Valerian (Valeriana officinalis) can be taken to gently relax muscles that may be excessively tense and painful. It can be taken as a tincture.

Nasal & Sinus Congestion

Nasal and sinus congestion can range from annoying runny noses due to a cold to intense throbbing pain from severe sinus congestion and infection. Appropriate remedies will correlate with the type of congestion.

Potential Root Causes

- Seasonal allergies
- Cold and flu
- Sinus infection
- Exposure to irritants
- Food intolerances and sensitivities

Minimalist Natural Medicine Cabinet Remedies

- Sea salt can be made into a saline solution and used as a nasal rinse 1-3 times a day to thin and eliminate mucus congestion. A pinch of baking soda can be added to the saline solution for extra comfort.
- Cold & Flu relief tea can be taken 1-3 times daily, especially if the congestion is due to infection.
- Elderberry syrup or gummies and echinacea extract can be taken if the congestion is due to infection.
- Garlic and ginger can be added liberally to the diet to help thin mucus secretions.
- Garlic can be finely minced and added to a spoonful of honey for children who dislike the taste of garlic on its own.
- Eucalyptus essential oil can be inhaled from a tissue, cotton ball, or directly from the bottle. It can also be diluted and used topically on the chest to help promote clear breathing and expel excess mucus. Lavender can be added for children and peppermint for older children and adults.

Specific Remedies

- Spicy foods, like garlic and ginger listed above, as well as horseradish, onions, and cayenne, can be added to the diet to help thin and expel congestion.
- Dairy can often cause chronic nasal congestion in people who have an intolerance. A dairy elimination diet can be trialed to see if congestion clears.

Nausea & Upset Stomach

Nausea is a very uncomfortable feeling, especially when it leads to vomiting. Though vomiting is sometimes inevitable and the quickest way to recover, some gentle remedies can help calm the stomach and alleviate nausea.

Potential Root Causes

- Infection
- Food poisoning
- Stress and anxiety
- Strong emotions, such as grief, nervousness, and worry

Minimalist Natural Medicine Cabinet Remedies

- Tummy Tea can be taken as a strong infusion while symptoms last.
- Ginger can be brewed into a strong infusion or decoction and taken while symptoms last. Ginger can also be cut into small pieces and candied to make a convenient nausea remedy.
- Apple cider vinegar can be added to water and sipped to reduce nausea and boost digestion. This can be helpful with nausea that follows eating.
- Lemon slices can be squeezed into water or herbal teas to add another stomach-calming flavor.
- Elderberry syrup or gummies can be taken if nausea is due to an infection.
- Relaxing Nervine Tea can be taken as a strong infusion if nausea is connected to stress or emotional upsets.
- Sweet orange and/or peppermint essential oils can be inhaled for 10-15 minutes, either directly from the bottle or from a cotton ball or tissue.

Specific Remedies

- Fennel seed can reduce nausea and upset stomach. It can be taken as an infusion or extract, or by simply chewing 3-5 whole fennel seeds.
- Herbal bitters can be taken before meals to promote good digestion if nausea happens at specific times of the day.

Poison Ivy/Oak/Sumac

Poison ivy, poison oak, and poison sumac grow all over the USA and other parts of the world. They produce a sticky, irritating oil called urushiol, and this oil causes a painful, itchy, blistering rash in most people.

Potential Root Causes
- Contact with urushiol

Minimalist Natural Medicine Cabinet Remedies
- Witch hazel can be applied topically over affected areas.
- Bentonite clay can be mixed into a paste with witch hazel and applied over the affected areas. Baking soda and/or sea salt can be added to the clay for additional relief.
- Baking soda can be added to warm bathwater to calm inflammation and itching.
- Apple cider vinegar can be applied topically over a stubborn rash that is slow to respond to witch hazel and bentonite clay.
- Aloe vera gel can be applied topically after applying witch hazel or apple cider vinegar and before applying bentonite clay paste. It can also be applied as the rash heals, before applying a healing salve.
- Peppermint essential oil can be diluted in a carrier oil and applied topically to reduce inflammation and itching. This is best done after the initial blistering has calmed and over unbroken skin.
- Healing salve can be applied over affected areas after the rash has dried up and begins to heal.
- Turmeric can be taken internally to reduce overall inflammation.

Specific Remedies

- Pink calamine lotion is another simple remedy that works well for poison ivy, poison oak, and poison sumac rashes.
- Severe reactions or those affecting internal tissues like the mouth, throat, and lungs should be seen by a medical professional.

Rashes

Rashes can be quite a mystery, especially with children. They can occur for a host of reasons and can be dry, like eczema, or weeping, like chickenpox. Some rashes itch, while others just look uncomfortable. Finding the root cause is the foundation of treating rashes longterm.

Potential Root Causes

- Chemical sensitivity
- Infection
- Food intolerances and sensitivities
- Contact irritation
- Gut flora imbalances (dysbiosis)

Minimalist Natural Medicine Cabinet Remedies

- Baking soda can be added to bathwater to reduce itching and inflammation.
- Bentonite clay can be made into a paste and spread over the affected area to dry up a weepy rash.
- Healing salve can be spread over the affected area if the rash is dry and inflamed.
- Aloe gel can be applied to irritated or dry rash areas.
- Lavender essential oil can be diluted in a carrier oil and applied topically. Tea tree oil can also be included with a total dilution ranging from 1-5 drops per teaspoon carrier, depending on the age of the person and size of the rash.
- Echinacea extract and/or elderberry syrup or gummies can be taken if the rash is due to viral infection.

Specific Remedies

- An elimination diet can uncover food sensitivities and intolerances if rashes appear regularly, especially on the cheeks.
- Eliminating artificial fragrances from personal care and cleaning products can eliminate rashes in some individuals.
- Probiotic supplements and/or fermented foods and drinks can restore healthy gut flora and reduce incidences of rashes, especially when the rashes occur after antibiotic use.
- Dandelion root (*Taraxacum officinale*) and milk thistle seed (*Silybum marianum*) can be taken to support the liver and natural detoxification.
- Oatmeal can be tied in a cloth or placed in a reusable tea bag, then added to bathwater to soothe dry, itchy rashes.

Sore Throat

A sore throat may be accompanied by a cough, but not always. It can be quite painful, especially if it is from an infection, and makes communicating in daily life difficult.

Potential Root Causes

- Infection
- Vocal strain
- Exposure to irritants
- Postnasal drip

Minimalist Natural Medicine Cabinet Remedies

- Honey can be taken by the teaspoonful to soothe irritated throat tissue.
- A simple anti-inflammatory, throat-soothing drink can be made by making a strong ginger infusion or decoction, then adding a teaspoon of honey and squeeze of lemon juice. This can be taken throughout the day.
- Cold & Flu Relief Tea can be taken throughout the day with honey if the sore throat is due to infection.
- Echinacea extract can be taken 3-5 times per day if the sore throat is due to infection.
- Elderberry syrup or gummies can be taken 3-5 times per day if the sore throat is due to infection.
- Garlic can be taken 3 times per day if the sore throat is due to infection.
- One teaspoon sea salt can be mixed with 1 cup warm water to form a strong saltwater gargle that can be used 1-3 times daily.

Specific Remedies

- Powdered slippery elm bark (*Ulmus rubra*) or marshmallow root (*Althaea officinalis*) can be made into a thick paste with honey, then rolled into lozenges about the size of a pinky finger's tip. These can be left out to dry for a day, then stored in the refrigerator and used as needed to soothe a painful throat.
- Mullein leaf (*Verbascum thapsus*) and licorice root (*Glycyrrhiza glabra*) can be taken as an infusion to soothe irritated throat tissue.
- Sore throat from a strep infection may require medical treatment and antibiotic therapy.

Stress & Anxiety

Stress is a part of everyday life, but when it becomes excessive or leads to anxiety, it becomes a problem. Herbal and aromatherapeutic remedies can provide some relief and help make stress more manageable.

Potential Root Causes

- Difficult seasons and situations
- Unresolved problems
- Worry, grief, fear, and other intense emotions

Minimalist Natural Medicine Cabinet Remedies

- Lavender and/or sweet orange essential oil can be deeply inhaled for 10-15 minutes, directly from the bottle or from a tissue or cotton ball.
- Epsom salt baths, with or without diluted essential oil, can reduce feelings of stress and improve sleep quality.
- Relaxing Nervine Tea can be taken as a strong infusion 1-3 times per day as needed.

Specific Remedies

- Lifestyle approaches, like appropriate exercise or activity, journaling, prayer, and time outdoors away from technology can help with stress management.
- Massage therapy can reduce stress levels and provide a needed, relaxing experience. Essential oils can be combined with massage for additional benefit.
- Vitamin D and omega 3 fatty acid supplementation can reduce feelings of stress and anxiety in some individuals, especially during months with cold weather and little sunshine.
- Adaptogenic herbs help the body respond to stress. These can be taken as tinctures and include the herbs ashwaganda (*Withania somnifera*), holy basil (*Ocimum sanctum*), reishi (*Ganoderma lucidum*), rhodiola (*Rhodiola rosea*), eleuthero (*Eleutherococcus senticosus*), and others.

Teething

Parents are often highly aware of when their babies and toddlers get new teeth because the little ones tend to sleep less and cry more. These young ones need the gentlest remedies that will provide some relief from the discomfort.

Potential Root Causes

- New teeth emerging

Minimalist Natural Medicine Cabinet Remedies

- Lavender essential oil can be diffused in a room for 15-30 minutes before the baby goes to sleep to promote relaxation. This is appropriate for babies 6 months old and older.
- Relaxing Nervine Tea can be made into a strong infusion, then small washcloths dipped in the infusion and placed in the freezer. Older babies and toddlers can chew on the washcloths, gaining relief from both the infusion and the cold.
- Breastfeeding mothers of young babies can drink the Relaxing Nervine Tea and pass the calming benefits on to their babies through breast milk.
- Lavender essential oil can be diluted in a carrier oil and applied along the jawline of older babies and toddlers. One drop of essential oil in 1-2 teaspoon(s) carrier oil is appropriate for babies 6 months old and older.

Specific Remedies

- Clove bud essential oil (*Syzygium aromaticum* flos) has analgesic properties and is often used to successfully relieve toothache pain. It requires careful diluting, though, as it can irritate gums if used too heavily. One drop of clove bud essential oil in 1 teaspoon food-grade carrier oil can be used on toddlers age 2 and above, applied to irritated gum tissue with a cotton swab.

Warts

Common warts result from skin infections with human papillomavirus strains. They're very common in children and tend to appear on the hands, elbows, and knees.

Potential Root Causes

- Exposure to HPV strain
- Weakened or developing immune system

Minimalist Natural Medicine Cabinet Remedies

- Apple cider vinegar can be applied topically every night by soaking small bits of cotton ball with the vinegar, then securing over the wart with an adhesive bandage. This can be repeated every night until the wart is removed. For young children with sensitive skin, apple cider vinegar can be diluted in equal parts water.
- Healing salve can be applied around warts during the apple cider vinegar treatment to protect the surrounding skin.
- Healing salve can be applied to the wart area once the wart has died out.
- Elderberry syrup or gummies can be taken daily for immune support.

Specific Remedies

- Zinc supplementation can improve immune function if warts are stubborn or tend to reappear.

Part 4:
Continued Learning

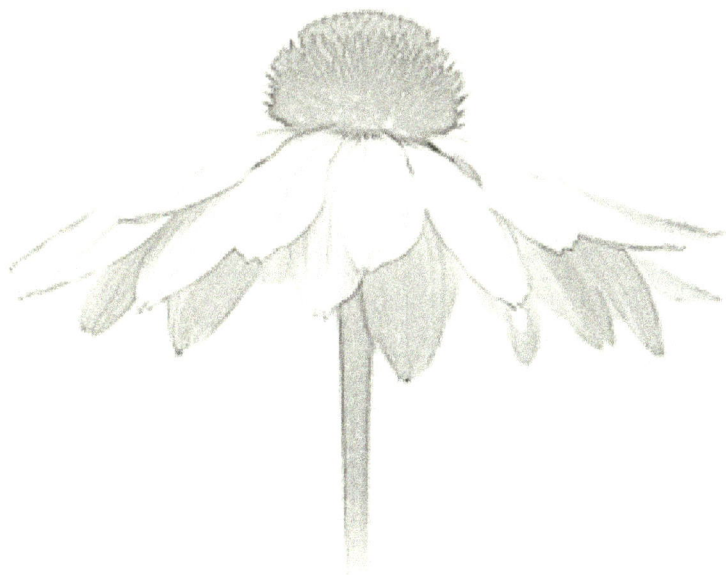

Final Encouragement

Even when stocking a Minimalist Natural Medicine Cabinet instead of an entire closet filled with remedies, you may still struggle to know where to start. Maybe the common kitchen ingredients and drugstore finds feel safe, but those few specialty purchases just seem too big. You might be worried about failing with even the simplest start.

Before you go any farther, give yourself permission to set aside the need to do it all and do it perfectly right away. Just start somewhere with one step forward.

Remember the goals behind a Minimalist Natural Medicine Cabinet? One of them is less stress and intimidation.

Start with what you already know. Then choose just one thing from the collection to add. Work with it for a few weeks or a few months, whatever it takes to feel confident with that remedy.

Then add another.

Continue that process until you've stocked the whole thing. By that time, you'll be ready to branch out to some of the Specific Remedies because you're no longer intimidated by the basics.

Eventually, you'll hardly need this guide because you'll have so much knowledge and experience backing you up.

But that all starts with just one step forward.

You can do it, and I'm cheering you on.

Oh, and when you have those exciting success moments? I'd love to hear about them. Email me (kristen@abetterwaytothrive.com) so I can celebrate with you.

Let's Connect

Exclusive Access & Subscriber Community

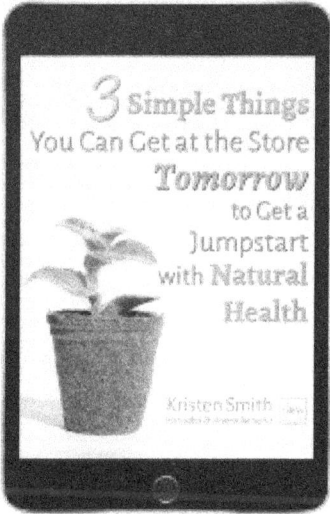

When you're ready to figure out the *hows* of natural health and finally make sense of herbs, essential oils, and healthy living in a way that honors your Christian faith, I invite you to join my free email community.

When you do, you'll get trusted guidance, practical help, and the reassurance you need to take smart steps toward thriving, natural health.

Subscribers get exclusive natural health content, insider updates and offers, and the opportunity to *just hit reply* and get a real answer back from me.

Plus, when you join, you'll get a free copy of my helpful guide *3 Things to Get at the Store Tomorrow to Get a Jump Start with Natural Living.*

Learn more and get your free guide here:
https://abetterwaytothrive.com/join

One-on-One Help

When you're facing a health challenge, the internet can be a wild place.

You can spend hours on Google search ater Google search, typing in all sorts of questions about natural remedies and getting enough diferent opinions to make your head swim.

But there's a better way.

When we work together, one-on-one, through my Thriving Health Consultations, you get to skip the confusion and enter into a partnership that gives you the confidence you need to move forward with your health.

As a trained herbalist, certified aromatherapist, and holistic health educator, I want to help make your natural health journey a little clearer and easier.

Because even though no one has all the answers for you and your health, having a trusted guide to point you in the right direction can do wonders.

If you're tired of wandering all over the internet, losing precious hours and energy trying to figure things out on your own, I'd love to talk with you.

Jessica said:

> *I was worried I would be judged for my choices, but Kristen helped me see that no one is perfect and change happens over time. I stopped beating myself up over all the things I thought I needed to do right away. Now that I can break down my big picture goal into manageable chunks, we have momentum to keep moving forward.*

Visit me here to learn more and get started:
https://abetterwaytothrive.com/services/
thriving-health-consultations

Keep Learning with Additional Resources

Once you master your Minimalist Natural Medicine Cabinet remedies, you might be ready to expand your natural health knowledge and add to your apothecary.

After joining my email community, the following resources will help you continue learning.

You can see them all at
https://abetterwaytothrive.com/shop

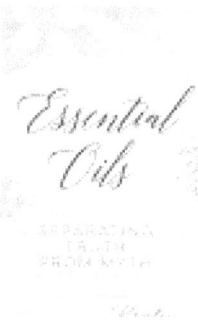

It can be really hard to know what to believe about essential oils. Set yourself up for better, safer results with this information-packed book that cuts through 25 common essential oil myths.

Get *Essential Oils: Separating Truth from Myth*, available on PDF, Kindle, and Paperback.

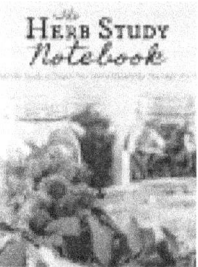

There are a lot of ways to learn about herbs, but one thing will help your learning really stick.

Discover how to spend time with one herb, learn it inside and out, and record all of your findings in one organized place you can go back to again and again with *The Herb Study Notebook*, a printable PDF.

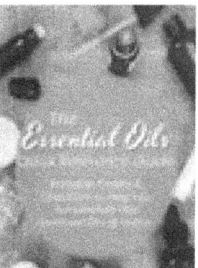

No matter how many times you use essential oils, there's a lot to remember. This printable set of smart charts and checklists puts all the information you need right at your fingertips.

The Essential Oils Quick Reference Guide makes using essential oils at home easier than ever!

Acknowledgments

First, thank you to my email community for their help with this project. Your feedback was invaluable! Leslie, Carolin, Sandy, Kari, Jennifer, Kendra, Stacie, Mary Lou, Tricia, Debra, Courtney, Linda, Tara, Uma, and the couple anonymous replies, I appreciate your extra interest and investment in this project. I hope it is a valuable asset in your home!

Thank you to my wonderful family for always supporting me in these projects. To my incredible crew of precious people, teaching you and caring for you is the most important work I'm blessed to do. Thank you for helping me set aside time and space to work, and for holding the baby while I did so. To Jesse, you're perfect for me and will always be my favorite. Thank you for believing in me, supporting me, and encouraging me. You're my guy and I'm honored to be your wife.

All praise and glory for these natural remedies belongs to the Creator God who loved us enough to provide remedies for our journey through this fallen world. *"For by Him were all things created, that are in heaven, and that are in earth, visible and invisible, whether they be thrones, or dominions, or principalities, or powers: all things were created by Him, and for Him: And he is before all things, and by Him all things consist."* Colossians 1:16-17

About the Author

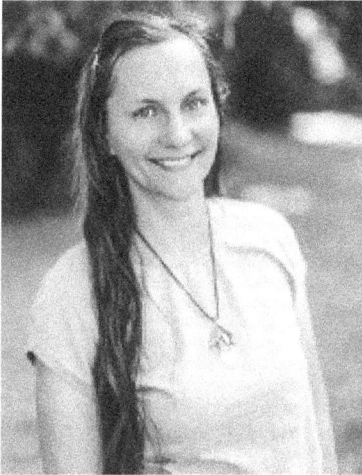

Kristen Smith is a trained herbalist and Certified Aromatherapist with multiple natural health certifications including Master Herbalist, Botanical Skincare, Aromatic Medicine, Holistic Wellness, and Professional Aromatherapy.

You can find her online at A Better Way to Thrive (abetterwaytothrive.com) where she can help you enjoy God's gift of natural health, one simple step at a time through free articles, helpful resources, and one-on-one consultations.

When you join her email community (https://abetterwaytothrive.com/join), you'll get the best of her content, plus exclusive bonuses that will keep you moving forward with herbs, essential oils, and other natural remedies. You'll also get her free guide *3 Things to Get at the Store Tomorrow to Get a Jumpstart with Natural Health*.

Though she loves her work, her home has her heart. She's married to Jesse, her high school sweetheart, and together they drive a huge van while raising a big family of sweet kiddos. They enjoy life in rural northeast Ohio, homeschooling and serving their local church in the pastoral role. Life is never dull, always busy, and most importantly, covered in God's grace. For that, she is eternally thankful.

To work individually with Kristen, schedule classes or speaking events, or with other inquiries, email her at kristen@abetterwaytothrive.com.

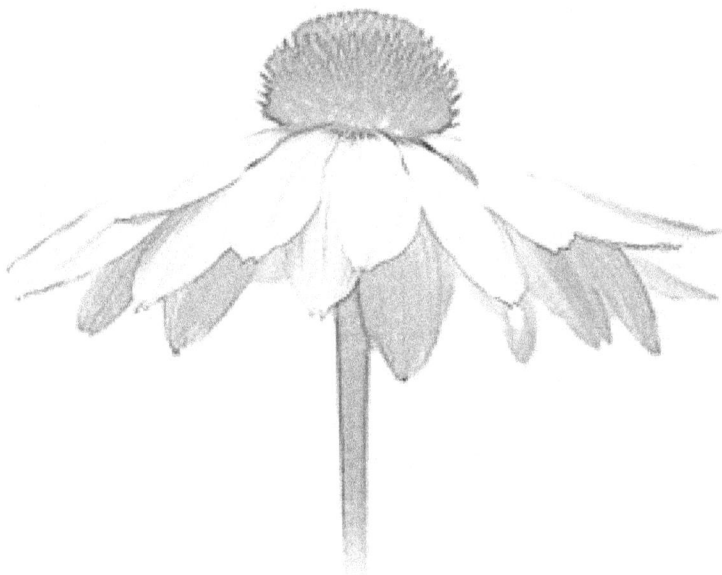

Learn more at

ABetterWayToThrive.com

www.ingramcontent.com/pod-product-compliance
Lightning Source LLC
Chambersburg PA
CBHW022100020426
42335CB00012B/760